Praise for Refram

"No one wins the shame game! The only way to win is to not play, and Irene Rollins will show you. All of us fight our own demons, but the enemy is a defeated foe. This is a timely message, and Irene is a prophetic voice."

—MARK BATTERSON, *NEW YORK TIMES* BESTSELLING AUTHOR, *THE CIRCLE MAKER*

"Compelling. Honest. Hopeful. Insightful. Helpful. Irene Rollins shares her powerful and inspiring journey through addiction while serving as a Christian leader. After hitting rock bottom, she has done the courageous and hard work of moving toward health and wholeness. She has much to teach us. No matter what you are struggling to overcome, this book can be a game changer and the path to a better future. As Irene says, 'recovery applies to everyone.'"

—LANCE WITT, FOUNDER OF REPLENISH MINISTRIES

"Irene has turned her biggest season of pain into her biggest source of purpose. Instead of allowing her past mistakes and regrets to turn into a prison of shame, she has turned them into a platform to help people around the world. This book is packed full of practical, inspirational, and helpful wisdom to help you do the same!"

—SHAWN JOHNSON, SENIOR PASTOR OF RED ROCKS CHURCH AND AUTHOR OF *ATTACKING ANXIETY*

"This is a right-book-at-the-right-time read! Sarah and I have been honored to walk with and watch Irene and Jimmy as they have walked this freedom journey over the last several years. This book captures it all perfectly! What a model and example the Rollins have become. I, along with so many people, need this book right now."

—MATT KELLER, FOUNDING AND LEAD PASTOR, NEXT LEVEL CHURCH, AND AUTHOR OF *GOD OF THE UNDERDOGS*

"Prepare to be blown away by Irene's testimony—her transparency opens the door to experience God's relentless love and passionate pursuit to free His people from shame. Irene invites you on her journey from addiction to recovery, brokenness to wholeness, and shame to joy. It is an invitation for anyone who feels alone to join her on the road back to the abundant life Jesus offers. I've had a front row seat to witness the miraculous transformation possible when we bravely face our fear and believe the truest thing about us is indeed what God says about us—now, this book is your front row seat."

—JULIE MULLINS, CO-SENIOR PASTOR OF
CHRIST FELLOWSHIP CHURCH

"We love Irene's courageous vulnerability with her story! The power of a leader standing up and being honest about their struggles and pain breaks down walls and makes it safe for others to admit they are hurting and struggling too. Through *Reframe Your Shame* Irene is revealing that addiction affects even those who appear to have their life together. As she walks us through her recovery process, she makes it safe for others to do so as well. Thank you, Irene, for recovering out loud so others don't have to struggle in silence!"

—JOHNNY AND JENI BAKER, PASTOR AND GLOBAL
CO-EXECUTIVE DIRECTORS OF CELEBRATE RECOVERY

"Raw. Determined. Authentic. Real. Those are just some of the words that come to mind when I think of my friend Irene. In her new book *Reframe Your Shame*, she shares with the world her story of over overcoming a seemingly impossible feat—breaking free from the grips of alcoholism. Irene's story gives readers confidence and courage to take bold steps that will allow them to reach freedom from their own shame."

—TIM TIMBERLAKE, PASTOR OF CELEBRATION CHURCH
AND AUTHOR OF *THE POWER OF 1440* AND *ABANDON*

Reframe Your Shame

Reframe Your Shame

EXPERIENCE FREEDOM FROM
WHAT HOLDS YOU BACK

IRENE ROLLINS

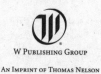

W PUBLISHING GROUP

AN IMPRINT OF THOMAS NELSON

Published in Nashville, Tennessee, by W Publishing, an imprint of Thomas Nelson.

Published in association with The Bindery Agency, www.TheBinderyAgency.com.

Thomas Nelson titles may be purchased in bulk for educational, business, fundraising, or sales promotional use. For information, please email SpecialMarkets@ThomasNelson.com.

Unless otherwise noted, Scripture quotations taken from The Holy Bible, New International Version®, NIV®. Copyright © 1973, 1978, 1984, 2011 by Biblica, Inc.® Used by permission of Zondervan. All rights reserved worldwide. www.Zondervan.com. The "NIV" and "New International Version" are trademarks registered in the United States Patent and Trademark Office by Biblica, Inc.®

Scripture quotations marked AMP are taken from the Amplified® Bible (AMP). Copyright © 2015 by The Lockman Foundation. Used by permission. www.Lockman.org.

Scripture quotations marked ESV are taken from the ESV® Bible (The Holy Bible, English Standard Version®). Copyright © 2001 by Crossway, a publishing ministry of Good News Publishers. Used by permission. All rights reserved.

Scripture quotations marked MSG are taken from THE MESSAGE. Copyright © 1993, 2002, 2018 by Eugene H. Peterson. Used by permission of NavPress. All rights reserved. Represented by Tyndale House Publishers, a Division of Tyndale House Ministries.

Scripture quotations marked NKJV are taken from the New King James Version®. Copyright © 1982 by Thomas Nelson. Used by permission. All rights reserved.

Scripture quotations marked NLT are taken from the Holy Bible, New Living Translation. Copyright © 1996, 2004, 2015 by Tyndale House Foundation. Used by permission of Tyndale House Ministries, Carol Stream, Illinois 60188. All rights reserved.

Scripture quotations marked NLV are taken from the New Life Version. Copyright © 1969, 2003 by Barbour Publishing, Inc.

Scripture quotations marked TLB are taken from The Living Bible. Copyright © 1971. Used by permission of Tyndale House Publishers, a Division of Tyndale House Ministries, Carol Stream, Illinois 60188. All rights reserved.

Scripture quotations marked TPT are taken from The Passion Translation®. Copyright © 2017, 2018 by Passion & Fire Ministries, Inc. Used by permission. All rights reserved. ThePassionTranslation.com.

This book is written as a source of information only. The information contained in this book should by no means be considered a substitute for the advice, decisions, or judgment of the reader's physician or other professional advisor. Readers who have issues with alcohol are urged to seek appropriate treatment.

Any internet addresses, phone numbers, or company or product information printed in this book are offered as a resource and are not intended in any way to be or to imply an endorsement by Thomas Nelson, nor does Thomas Nelson vouch for the existence, content, or services of these sites, phone numbers, companies, or products beyond the life of this book.

ISBN 978-0-7852-9004-9 (Audio)
ISBN 978-0-7852-9003-2 (eBook)
ISBN 978-0-7852-8982-1 (TP)

Library of Congress Control Number: 2022001414

ISBN 978-0-7852-8982-1

Printed in the United States of America

22 23 24 25 26 LSC 10 9 8 7 6 5 4 3 2 1

To the Rollins Crew
Jimmy, Kayla, Jaden, and Maya.
Thank you for doing the work, listening, and
empathizing, for being amazing forgivers, and for loving
me past my yuck. I love you with all my heart.
Rollins five forever.

Contents

CONTENTS

PART 3: DO THE WORK
A Framework for Getting Healthy and Managing a Healthier Way of Life

Foreword

*I*rene and I had our first meal together at Applebee's in Pennsylvania. No, it wasn't fancy (unless you *love* Applebee's, and then of course it was), but it *was* a meal laden with destiny.

Listen, I had fangirled over Irene from afar for years. I'd heard her speak alongside her husband Jimmy about the good work they were doing in Baltimore at the time, and I wanted to pick her brain, glean from her, and simply sit with her. Truthfully, I wanted to be her friend. Little did I know, she'd recently read my first book, *She Is Free*, and put meeting me on her list of goals for that year. When she heard I was speaking a mere two-hour drive away from her home at a mutual friend's church, she got in a car, made the trip, and sat herself in the front row. I couldn't believe my eyes when I saw her sitting there. We both knew we had to share a meal together that evening.

That night in Pennsylvania was the beginning of a friendship that would change both of our lives. We'd speak at conferences together, have long chats on the phone, celebrate together, text check-ins, encouragements, voice memos, and so much more. One of my favorite memories was surprising Irene to celebrate that she had achieved five years of sobriety! When she came around the corner of her home and saw her friends quietly waiting, tucked away in the living room ready to surprise her... well, the look of shock and joy on her face will forever be a sweet memory for me.

Little did I know how much I wouldn't just love being her friend, but I would need her friendship through some of my toughest years of leading and simply living life as a human on planet earth. It's no joke down here. We need Jesus and we deeply need one another. Yes, I had written the book *She Is Free*, but there were still parts of my life that needed healing. Areas that were too intimate and scary to share with just anyone. Luckily, Irene had shown me the power of going first. Going first in being vulnerable. Going first in opening her life up for others. Going first in making a way.

The truth is we all need a friend unafraid of the dark night of our souls. And in a season where I was utterly shattered by certain circumstances that had become major pain points in my leadership life, Irene didn't look away nor shame me when I confessed my true state. She came alongside my bruised and battered soul, opened a door, and showed me the road to recovery.

I remember the day my husband said to me, "I think you need to call Irene and tell her everything." I mean, I knew I had a glaring need to break some cycles, and a man can only hear the same thing so many times, but I was so nervous to call Irene.

With my heart thumping in my chest, ears ringing in muffled tones, and my breath pumping in and out of my lungs at near panic attack rates, I dialed her number, and in an age where it usually goes to voicemail (that none of us actually listen to—because texting), she answered, "Hello friend..." and I broke. I poured out my soul, my fears, my pain, my struggle, and she didn't look away; she began to help me *reframe my shame*. She saw me, truly saw me, and spoke life.

One of my favorite lines to quote from Irene is, "Be authentic with the many and vulnerable with a few." She's one from my very small circle of friends that get to see all of me. The good, the bad, and the ugly. She said, "Well Andi, you're going to be okay, *and* we need a game plan." She jumped in like a good friend and coach, holding my feet to the fire. I then chose to keep showing up for my life, admitting and accepting my state before God, along with doing the work to walk in freedom. There was prayer, counseling, recovery, and accountability. I will say this: we're as accountable as we want to be. Even Irene couldn't force me to make changes or open up and tell the truth, but she was willing to walk with me.

Here's what you need to know as you read each page in this book: Irene does the work in her own life. She lives this. She hasn't simply jotted down a few ideas for you to add to a repertoire of knowledge; oh no, she has fought for her freedom and still contends for the ground she has yet to take. And when the giants show up, this powerful woman gets out her slingshot and calls in the reinforcements to come alongside her. Irene doesn't isolate herself. She chooses to reach out, tell the truth, and open up. She does the hard things. She continues to take the narrow road.

I'll never forget sitting in my home in Brooklyn a couple of years back with Jimmy and Irene dreaming and brainstorming the very heart of this book you now hold in your hands. Please understand that every word you read was fought for—many of them with tears. Irene is a warrior and a friend. This book will search your heart and bring you to your knees. I can pretty much guarantee you'll be inspired to make brave choices and do even braver things that change the trajectory of your life. It will cause you to admit, confess, and accept where you are before Jesus, and then do the work to *reframe your shame* in the hands of a loving God. Irene will be a faithful friend on every single page, going first, and opening a door to freedom for you to walk right through, just like she did for me.

Love,

Andi

Author of *She is Free, Fake or Follower,* and *Friendship—It's Complicated*

Introduction

My drinking career started when I was first introduced to alcohol at age ten. Unbeknownst to my parents, I helped myself to my dad's beautiful brown bottles of Guinness stout beer, which for some reason I thought was full of the vitamins I needed. Crazy, right? That first drink went down cold. I loved the burn, and I didn't hate the taste—even more, I loved the way it made me feel minutes later. *These vitamins must be good, because I sure do feel great!* I thought to myself.

At the time, we lived in Cameroon in West Africa, where my dad would get Guinness by the crate. So there was plenty around, and he didn't notice how quickly I depleted his stores. Little did I realize how I was altering my brain chemistry at a critical stage of my brain development. I became a little alcoholic. Boarding school in Switzerland at age fourteen made it worse because grabbing a six-pack was easy, with no drinking-age restriction that I was aware of at the time. I drank more and realized my high tolerance made me cool with my peers. As a teenager, going to bars and getting someone to buy me a drink was simple. And when I drank, *I drank a lot*, often blacking out.

Alcoholism is a sneaky and insidious disease. Not one of us is exempt from falling into addiction to a substance, person, or thing that is so brutally addictive in nature. Society tells us that drinking, staying in dysfunctional relationships, overworking to avoid real life, needing people's approval to function in life, overeating, and treating ourselves to calm anxiety and stress are all normal things to do. If we choose to live differently, those around us can make us feel like we're the odd ones out, or that something is wrong with us. Life gets hard, too, and a drink here and there to calm our nerves, to take the edge off our stress, can seem like a perfectly sensible thing to do. Avoiding conflict, as well as personal and relational issues, is also a regular practice for most adults.

I get it. I have been there. *You are not alone.*

Maybe you can identify with exposure to alcohol at a young age. Perhaps for you, your addiction was pornography, pain pills, perfectionism, or codependency. Maybe it began with exposure in your formative years as well. Whatever your coping mechanism of choice, an addiction was born, and you started down a path you would later regret, just as I did. All these experiences we had as young adults shape our lives over the years and decades to come.

Here's the good news that I want to share with you over the course of this book: God wants to turn your story around for your good, and for the good of others. He promises us in Romans 8:28 that He will turn *all* things around for the good of those who love Him and are called to His purpose. His purpose is for us to overcome our past, live free from the bondage that held us back, and step into a fulfilling life of true joy and freedom. This is attainable when we learn to reframe the way we look at our past experiences and our problems.

To reframe a situation simply means to see it from a different point of view. When you feel triggered, stuck, or confused, reframing helps you see the situation more constructively and problem solve, make decisions, and learn from your experiences rather than feel defeated by them.

When we embrace the idea that we have the power and wonderful opportunity to change the lens through which we view our lives, when we reframe the shame of our history, story, and problems, we are empowered to have them work for us rather than against us. It is never too late to change the trajectory of our lives and redirect the outcome of our stories. The mistakes we see as failures can be reframed, and we can learn to see them as opportunities for growth and development. Failure occurs when we don't learn from our mistakes but allow them to define or defeat us. Reframing, however, empowers us to grow, heal, recover, experience less anxiety, and even get better results in treatment of addiction and mental health challenges. Reframing improves our quality and enjoyment of life in general. When our mindset changes, our behavior changes as well. My hope is that by the time you reach the end of this book, you will see what you thought was your greatest shame reframed into your greatest purpose. That you will see God working "all things" out for your good!

PART I

Admit

The Journey of Addiction

CHAPTER 1

How Did I Get Here?

I *didn't even see it coming.*

From the outside, my life looked pretty close to perfect. In my early thirties, I was married to my pastor husband, had three kids and two dogs, and owned a home and two cars. I was a pastor leading an incredible growing and thriving church ministry located just south of Baltimore, Maryland, called i5 City with my husband, Jimmy. For me, this might as well have been the two-story home with the white picket fence, because everywhere I looked, I saw everything I'd ever dreamed.

Yet I wondered, *Shouldn't I be happier?* When I thought about the perfect life, we'd basically achieved that dream. Sure, our marriage could use some work, but it seemed like I couldn't fix it, so I decided, *It is what it is.* After all, I tried so hard to fix myself like any good Christian woman should, right? I thought I had to "have it all together." I couldn't let people see me sweat or see me cry or see that I felt miserable with a deep sorrow I couldn't explain. I didn't know what to do because I'd internalized the false, external expectation that my job as a woman, wife, pastor, and mom was to keep it all together. Why couldn't I feel the joy and peace I read about in the Bible? Why didn't I experience intimacy with God or with my husband, Jimmy, the way I saw other people around me genuinely experiencing those things? Why did it feel like I hit a wall with my ability to parent and connect emotionally with my then fourteen- and eleven-year-old daughters and thirteen-year-old son?

Why did I still have an aching inside me?

I was falling apart on the inside. I didn't have it all together. I felt like a fake, but I was exhausted trying to be there for everyone else while I struggled with the stress of pretending my life was perfect. *Who was I anyway? Who was I outside of what I did professionally? Who was I outside of the tasks I performed in my home?* The insecurity ate away at me daily, and I had no idea from where my deeply rooted anxiety was coming from. I had yet to identify the source, nor did I know how to address it. How could I even begin to articulate what was happening in my mind and body? Opening up honestly about my life and my pain was not a skill I had at the time.

I have come to find out that just because you pray a prayer and come into relationship with Jesus, the Son of the living God, doesn't mean all your problems go away. But the desire to be perfect continued to gnaw at me. All my years in church gave me a long list of things to do to flourish in my life. Faithfully, I did them all, believing they would work. I went to church regularly, loved on the people there, and supported my husband wholeheartedly. I went to counseling to work on myself. We went to marriage counseling and marriage retreats together. I prayed, read my Bible, and devoured every self-help book known to man.

Ultimately, I fell into a "try hard, *try harder*, and eventually give up" cycle. Have you ever felt like that—completely blindsided by life, by people, or even by yourself? If you've been there, if you are there, you are not alone. Perhaps like me, you get up, go through the motions, pretend you're okay, and hope for change but feel helpless to make the changes you want to see. I felt hopeless at times. Would anything ever change? But secretly I wondered, *Is this my life sentence? Will I just live on autopilot, doing and doing and doing and taking care of everyone but myself until the day I die?*

Do you realize that the things we hope, believe, pray for, and receive can also cause stress in our lives? I wish someone had dropped that gold nugget of wisdom into my life a lot sooner. Many people, women especially, feel guilty when they struggle to cope with and live the life they thought they wanted. Intuitively, we know that relationships are challenging, parenting isn't easy, and managing households and careers is difficult. But we feel bad for feeling bad. Most of us do not possess healthy coping skills or know how to process stress in our lives, so we hide our struggles. We become bound by shame, and shame produces isolation and silence. Then we try to keep everything inside—except that's impossible, so we find other ways to deal with the pain we feel.

I'm a Recovering Alcoholic

In 2017 the National Survey on Drug Use and Health found that twenty million Americans ages twelve and older battled a substance abuse disorder of some kind. Seventy-four percent of those surveyed defined alcohol as their

> Do you realize that the things we hope, believe, pray for, and receive can also cause stress in our lives?

struggle. That same year, 9.5 million American adults also suffered from a mental illness, alongside their addiction.[1] People across multiple sectors of society, including people in church pews and on church platforms, are struggling with substance abuse.

The Barna Group produced a study in 2017 called "The State of Pastors," consisting of data from over fourteen thousand interviews across forty denominations. While their findings disclosed some positive trends, the report also revealed that one in five pastors struggles with an addiction and 40 percent deal with depression; more than half shared that the ministry takes a significant toll on their marriages and families. Female pastors, making up just 9 percent of senior pastors (although 9 percent is triple the percentage from twenty-five years ago), feel greater scrutiny, loneliness, and isolation from people than their male counterparts.[2] I am among the twenty million Americans struggling with an addiction and among the one in five pastors wrestling with a destructive habit, one that hurt me and my family.

I couldn't wait to unwind from the day with a glass (or two or three) of wine. Without really understanding why, I would do anything to take the edge off. Subtly, and then suddenly, alcohol became my go-to, my comfort, and my relief. Underneath the stress, I felt the (perceived) expectations from family, ministry, and my own impossible standards, all of which weighed on me constantly. Do you know what it's like to feel as though you're failing all the time? I drank to avoid not being perfect, to avoid feeling like I had failed everyone in my life. The hidden grief in my life, which I will share as we journey together in this book, lurked right beneath the surface. Alcohol helped me cope and hide from the fears and stresses of abandonment, rejection, loss, transition, and failure, all of which I was not yet ready to face.

What's Underneath Your Stress?

Research tells us that the top five stressors in life are (1) the death of a loved one, (2) job loss or job change, (3) moving (or buying a home), (4) getting married or divorced, and (5) some kind of major illness.[3] It's easy to look back now and see exactly how alcohol became my way of dealing with any kind of major stress. At times, I faced all five of these major stressors at the same time.

Jimmy and I bought and sold several homes while raising our family and made job changes that involved key family members, which complicated things to another degree. Then we suffered a string of losses, including the sudden tragic death of my brother in 2003 and then my father in 2007, along with the deaths of friends in our church (some of whom were children or young adults), along with other losses in my husband's family. Each loss was followed by the fatigue of grief that left us aching, empty, and numb. All of this occurred on top of transitioning our church from the original pastors, my husband's parents, to our leadership. Plus, ordinary life kept happening—as it does for everyone.

I had no training on how to walk through grief or the fatigue of constant loss, stress, and transition. Even with my shelf of self-help books, lots of prayer, and doing all the right things a Christian should do, I could not find a way forward.

How did I get here? I wondered.

The introduction of alcohol when I was young was not just a taste here and there. I abused it—when I drank, I drank a lot. For me, just a buzz wasn't appealing or worthwhile. In my mind, the purpose of drinking alcohol was to get drunk. What other reason was there to drink besides escaping reality? Besides, alcohol helped me loosen up and get brave enough to be the person I could not be when I was sober. Drinking alcohol helped me feel confident, like I fit in, and gave me a sense of belonging. I relaxed enough to be less inhibited at parties and in social settings. Alcohol helped me temporarily get past my insecurity that I was not and never would be enough.

At the time, I thought it was fun to seemingly transcend the problems of the world and enter a false reality that was void of issues, pain, and problems. Problem was, once I woke up with a vicious hangover, I was miserable and often felt disgusted with myself and full of shame from my behaviors and things I allowed myself to do while drunk. This fueled my anxiety, insecurity, and negativity toward myself and sent me down a slippery slope of depression. I often wondered if this was all there was to life. Go to work and/or school, drink myself into oblivion, wake up hung over, then wait for the next opportunity to repeat it. This was the sad reality of my early drinking days.

However, between age twenty-one and thirty-two, I didn't drink a drop. Meeting Jimmy had radically changed my life and everything I did (or didn't do), including drinking alcohol. I belonged to a family, and I started popping out babies all through my twenties, so I lived off that adrenaline high for some time. I felt like I was experiencing true happiness, but it didn't last once the thrill of the childbirth experience ended when I had my last child at age twenty-eight. The emptiness inside my soul continued to grow as I dug deep into performing and doing and white-knuckling through life, making busyness and achievement my goal for satisfaction and self-worth. I never said out loud that I missed having alcohol in my life; I just prayed for the desire to go away, and for the most part it did. But secretly, I longed for the numbness that alcohol brought me.

I was thirty-two when I reintroduced alcohol into my life. My husband and I made the fateful decision to drink on a vacation together in 2009. We didn't think it was a big deal to drink in moderation, and my guard was down. We vacationed in a city away from the pressures of ministry and away from anyone who knew us. But what I meant for vacation, and perhaps occasionally on weekends, slowly became something I anticipated every single day. Alcohol became my stress reliever. As soon as I walked in the door from a hard, long day at work, I found myself unintentionally pouring a glass of wine.

The apostle Paul, a man who also understood the impact of the culture around him on his own life, as well as the transformative power of Christ, wrote this:

> And so, dear brothers and sisters, I plead with you to give your bodies to God because of all he has done for you. Let them be a living and holy sacrifice—the kind he will find acceptable. This is truly the way to worship him. Don't copy the behavior and customs of this world, but let God transform you into a new person by changing the way you think. Then you will learn to know God's will for you, which is good and pleasing and perfect. (Romans 12:1–2 NLT)

Similar to the culture Paul lived in, our culture sends the message that alcohol is okay. What's the big deal with having a drink anyway? I even bought a T-shirt that read: Will Run for Wine. Even more, I started to become a wine connoisseur, which I thought was rather classy. Besides, Jesus turned water into wine, right? I felt more grown-up and unbound by the fundamentalist "religious" thing that told me there was something wrong with drinking.

Nobody was going to tell me what to do or how to do it. I enjoyed having a margarita at Mexican restaurants. I love chips and salsa, and I used that excuse to go to Mexican restaurants just so I could get a margarita. Eventually, I began to add an extra shot or two of tequila in my margaritas. *I just have a high tolerance*, I reasoned, without even considering that I was conforming to the behaviors and customs of this world.

The idea that our culture celebrates drinking (and other addictions too) worked for me, because I wanted to drink. And the social stigma I felt in the church when I was younger evaporated in a culture that accepted (even approved of) dependency on alcohol. I didn't realize that I was developing a "need" for it over time, but before I knew it, a drink helped me calm my nerves and ease into the evening every single night. I became a "take the edge off–aholic." My religious background influenced me to believe that pastors can't be seen drinking or getting drunk in public, so happy hour needed to happen at home for me unless I was able to find a restaurant off the beaten path where I didn't think I would run into anyone from our congregation. I assumed I would be looked down upon and judged if I was seen drinking in public, and I resented the fact that I felt like I had to hide it. The pattern of hiding my drinking was only perpetuated by this belief I made up in my own mind that I could not drink in public.

I love *The Message* version of Romans 12:2: "Don't become so well-adjusted to your culture that you fit into it without even thinking. Instead, fix your attention on God. You'll be changed from the inside out. Readily recognize what he wants from you, and quickly respond to it. Unlike the culture around you, always dragging you down to its level of immaturity, God brings the best out of you, develops well-formed maturity in you."

Adjusting to our culture is so easy that most of us try to fit in without even thinking about it. This happens to all of us in some way. Culture is always shaping us. Beth Moore wrote in her *Daniel* Bible study that if we are not actively fighting the indoctrination of culture, we are actively being indoctrinated by it.[4] As I write this chapter, there is a reckoning happening in our nation over the issue of racism. Until 2021, many people, especially Christians, did not understand how much implicit racism was entrenched in their lives, workplaces, and churches. Without even knowing it, we can "sneeze" racism. Just as a sneeze is caused by irritation in our bodies (specifically, nasal passages), impelling us to involuntarily and convulsively expel air through the nose and mouth, we react similarly with irritations in our culture that disrupt our normalcy.

Even our varied responses to the COVID-19 pandemic is telling. People have had explosive, even automatic reactions about what they believe is right or wrong, about how we should handle vaccinations or whether we should wear masks or not. Opinions are shared or reposted on social media without so much as a thought or evaluation of how it may affect others. People of influence use their platforms to voice opinions that create confirmation bias for people living in a culture full of fear and uncertainty, further exacerbating the fear.

These sometimes volatile and harsh opinions have caused division in our communities. If we do not take the time to evaluate the basis of our beliefs through the lens of the Bible and use the Word as our filter for handling difficulties, instead of what the culture around us is saying is the right or wrong way to handle things, we, too, can get caught up in conforming to culture. We, too, can be at risk of allowing culture to dictate our reality. We absorb fear by watching the news, and we may subconsciously take on the biases of our upbringing, our communities, the news pundits we watch, and the articles and posts we read. If we're not careful, we become more acquainted with the way of our culture than we are with the way of Jesus.

As culture pertains to alcohol, drinking is considered "normal." In fact, turning twenty-one is a milestone in which we celebrate turning the legal drinking age. For me, it just signified not sneaking around anymore, because by the time I was twenty-one, I had already abused alcohol in such a way that it was no longer so appealing when I was allowed to drink legally. Drinking is socially acceptable at celebrations and for stress relief. It's the cool thing to do. In fact, it's rare to go anywhere without the opportunity to drink, and if you don't drink, it seems that there's something wrong with you. It's easy to ignore the telltale signs that we are, as Whoopi Goldberg says in the movie *Ghost*, "in danger, girl."[5]

Privately, my dependency continued to grow. I drank when I was cooking because it made meal preparation so much more fun, I thought. At least until I started burning things and forgetting ingredients, which of course my husband noticed. *What is the big deal about alcohol anyway?* I complained to him. *Why do you pressure me about how much I drink? I'm not hurting anyone.* At every turn, I justified my drinking, remaining in denial about how much I drank and how often. I refused to acknowledge that I drank every single day. I missed all the warning signs. On the nights I drank too much, I'd find an excuse to explain my behavior to myself, even while those nights became more and more frequent.

Like every addict, whether it is watching a little porn, doing some drugs, or overeating to process feelings, I thought I could control it. With minimal guilt, I allowed myself to binge without admitting that my life was becoming unmanageable and the consequences increasing. When I drank too much, I would tell myself it was just an accident, that it wouldn't happen again. *Don't I deserve to let loose from time to time?* I'd reason. *I'm a grown woman!*

When I found myself a little tipsy or Jimmy asked me how much I'd been drinking, I'd tell him that maybe I didn't eat enough that day. He soon got tired of my lame excuses.

There are more ways to access a good feeling than being inebriated. The crash of the day after never fixes the cause from the day before. I didn't know I was addicted until I tried to stop. I know that I can never touch alcohol again. My body chemistry is changed forever because I was in full-blown dependency on alcohol. That is the thing about dependency on a drug—we pick up right where we left off when we start up again. If I was abusing alcohol to the extent of blacking out, experiencing memory loss, putting stress on relationships, isolating myself, and rationalizing my drinking, that is where I would start off again.

Addiction Is for "Those People"

Sometimes we can create a caricature of the addict in our minds, but it's rarely an accurate picture. In doing so, we judge addicts as men and women making poor choices, having difficulty managing their lives, or choosing to hold a victim mentality. By imagining the absolute extremes of addiction, it becomes easy to write off people who struggle or to consider those who are honest about their addictions as weak. Such thinking allows us to overlook our own vulnerability to similar struggles.

Your struggle may not be with alcohol; instead, it might be with something that on the surface seems okay. We can develop an addiction to almost anything—money, security, work, achievements, social media, pride, others' approval, a need to be needed, control of romantic relationships, food, violence, pornography, sex, video games, media and entertainment, drugs, alcohol, or even our phones. All these things can be means of numbing ourselves for hours at a time.

By quickly judging addicts for extreme addictions, we can easily overlook our own struggles. How do I know this? Because I ignored the warning signs in my own life: rationalizing my behavior despite the increasing consequences, hiding my drinking, and isolating myself so no one would know the deep shame and remorse I felt. How did it get so easy to ignore those flashing red lights? It's different for everyone. Daily life, anxiety, depression, the pain of our past, and even the culture in which we live can all become overwhelming, so much so that ignoring the warnings becomes easier than acknowledging what's happening.

Often we simply don't want to think about the warning signs happening all around us. Thinking about pain hurts. Autopilot is so much easier. And human beings have the unique propensity to avoid pain, running away from it rather than toward it. We struggle to admit we need help, let alone to ask someone for it. The ability to think about what we're doing and the consequences of our actions is a prerequisite to dealing with our pain and considering change. With a brain hijacked by alcohol, I wasn't able to acknowledge my pain or make a change early on.

What Are the Warning Signs?

Let's look at three warning signs of an unhealthy habit or addiction. Think about your life. Do you see yourself in my struggle?

Perhaps it's not alcohol for you, but are you dealing with any of the following warning signs for some other unhealthy struggle in your life?

Rationalizing

Have you found yourself making excuses for why you do what you do? Saying aloud all the excuses you make up to explain why you did something you know was beyond moderation can sound crazy. Could it be that you're shopping so much that your house looks like you're hoarding an entire store? Are your credit cards maxing out, or are you piling up more debt than you can handle on your fixed income? Are you hopping from one relationship to another, finding yourself sad when you're single because you derive worth and value from others? Are you using food to deal with your emotions? Do you find yourself reasoning, *What's the big deal with just needing a little something to take the edge off each night?* And is the frequency increasing?

> Human beings have the unique propensity to avoid pain, running away from it rather than toward it.

If you answered yes to any of the above questions, you may be falling into a trap. I know that while under the influence, I was unable to reason properly. Rationalizing our behavior, even with the best excuses we can come up with, is a red flag we need to confront.

TAKE A MOMENT TO REFLECT: Is there a habit you are justifying to yourself and those around you? What is it?

Hiding

As a child, I excelled at hide-and-seek. I was a fast runner, stealthy, light on my feet, and small enough to hide in the most obscure hiding spaces. My talent for hiding clearly carried over into adulthood.

I transitioned from a regular drinker to a problem drinker when I began hiding how much I actually drank. Sneaking a glass here or a shot there without anyone noticing was too easy. I had no idea that the more I drank, the more I hid, and the more I binged and abused alcohol, the more dependent I became.

I felt extreme shame and remorse the morning after I binged and abused alcohol, which made me hide more. This is often what we do when we feel shame. Adam and Eve did it in the garden of Eden after deciding not to heed the wisdom God gave them about not eating fruit from a particular tree in the garden. They ate the fruit anyway and immediately felt shame because their eyes were opened to good and evil. So they hid from God. Genesis 3:8 says, "Then the man and his wife heard the sound of the LORD God as he was walking in the garden in the cool of the day, and they hid from the LORD God among the trees of the garden."

As with Adam and Eve, hiding increases our dependency on ourselves and forces us to turn to unhealthy coping mechanisms. Secrets make us sick with shame, and we run from the people, and the God, who can help us. Shame and resentment filled me after I drank, and then I looked to place blame somewhere to deflect it from myself. I blamed Jimmy and the church people for my hiding. Believing it was their fault that I had to sneak around made it easier to cope with the extreme shame I was experiencing for hiding my drinking. When we cannot admit we have a problem, we blame other people.

> **TAKE ANOTHER MOMENT TO REFLECT:** Is there a behavior you hide from the people who love you most? Do you feel shame or remorse and tell yourself the lie that you will never do it again?

Isolating

After rationalizing our decisions and hiding our behavior, we might begin to isolate ourselves. In isolation, it's easier to believe the lies that we are safe and under control, and that people can't reject us if they don't know the truth. I began to disconnect from my family, making Jimmy the bad guy and finding ways to be around my kids but not really present with them. At church on Sundays, I'd arrive on time and leave early, lessening my connection and presence with the congregation. Nobody could get too close to me, and I kept it that way on purpose. Distancing myself from others meant I was safe to continue drinking, and to remain isolated from them meant I didn't have to be honest about my life, my issues, and my pain. Isolation is a red flag begging for our attention.

> **TAKE A FINAL MOMENT TO CONSIDER:** Have you pushed loved ones away? Are you believing the lie that remaining isolated will keep you safe?

Reflect

Do you see yourself or a loved one in the story I've just shared? Are you ignoring the warning signs? Are you googling questions like "Am I an alcoholic?" Are you wondering if you have a problem with [fill in the blank]? Are you miserable, waking up sad, but still unable to stop doing the very thing you said you wouldn't do? What would it take for you to acknowledge and admit your pain? Dr. Henry Cloud, in his book *Boundaries with Kids*, wrote, "We change our behavior when the pain of staying the same becomes greater than the pain of changing. Consequences give us the pain that motivates us to change."[6] This is so true! Do you eat, drink, shop, smoke, gamble, overwork, or shame yourself in excess? Are you at the place yet where you want to spare yourself worse consequences, and you have the willingness or desire to stop? Ask yourself some questions to assess whether you or a loved one may have an issue with abuse of a substance.

Imagine asking yourself the following questions about whatever is out of moderation in your life that you may be "using," whether it is a substance (illegal drugs, alcohol, prescription drugs, food), person (obsession over a person or being in a relationship), thing, or even an activity (overworking, achieving, shopping, gambling). Replace the word "drinking" with your word.

In the past year, have you done any of the things listed below?

- Had times when you ended up drinking more or longer than you intended?
- More than once wanted to cut down or stop drinking or tried to but couldn't?
- Spent a lot of time drinking? Or being sick or getting over the aftereffects?
- Experienced a strong need or urge to drink?
- Found that drinking or being sick from drinking often

interfered with taking care of your home or family? Or caused job troubles or school problems?

- Continued to drink even though it was causing trouble with your family or friends?
- Given up or cut back on activities that were important or interesting to you or gave you pleasure, in order to drink?
- More than once gotten into situations while or after drinking that increased your chances of getting hurt or hurting others (such as driving, swimming, using machinery, walking in a dangerous area, or having unsafe sex)?
- Continued to drink even though it was making you feel depressed or anxious or adding to another health problem? Or after having had a memory blackout?
- Had to drink much more than you once did to get the effect you want? Or found that your usual number of drinks had much less effect than before?
- Found that when the effects of alcohol were wearing off, you had withdrawal symptoms, such as trouble sleeping, shakiness, irritability, anxiety, depression, restlessness, nausea, or sweating? Or sensed things that were not there?

Friend, I sincerely hope that the consequences of your addiction do not become as dire as mine before you decide to make a change. My journey to rock bottom and almost losing everything that was important to me, including the people I loved most in my life, took a swift turn down the slippery slope of addiction when I picked my drinking back up at age thirty-two and ended up in rehab six years later at age thirty-eight. It crept up on me slowly, without my seeing it coming, and almost destroyed my life. No matter what you've already done or whatever consequences you are facing, I want you to know there is a future and a hope for you. You are not alone in your struggles, and I believe this book will help you be more honest, get help, and step out of denial and shame into recovery on the road to freedom.

CHAPTER 2

Hiding, Performing, and Pretending

*H*ave you ever done something that shocked you? Have you become someone you don't recognize? Probably! You're human. At some point over a lifetime, you've likely felt this way about yourself. And there's probably not one specific event that led to this. Slowly, over time, one small decision after another led you to do the thing you thought you'd never do or to become the person you didn't mean to become. We don't intend to become a parent who screams at her kids or a friend who is consistently unable to show up for others, or a person who is not okay unless everyone else is okay. Life happens to us, and the way we respond is determined by our history and our sense of safety in relationships.

Maybe you have no idea what it means to be safe in relationships. Safety is a baseline for healthy connection and attachment to others that is developed in early childhood relationships with caretakers. When the early connections with parents or caretakers offer security, nurturing, and safety, we grow into secure adults able to connect authentically and show up as who we are. Without security, nurturing, and safety, we might hide our true selves and our feelings, pretend we are someone we are not, or perform our way into approval, connection, and achievement because this was safe and became a way to survive when feeling insecure. I know this from personal experience. But I didn't know another way. All I knew was that I was in pain, and I wanted it to stop. I wanted to overcome the pain of my past, but I thought that if I acknowledged it and tried to deal with it, the pain might kill me. How could I share with another human being how miserable I was in my marriage and that unthinkable things had stolen my innocence in my early childhood? The pain of hiding that I had been sexually abused was too much to acknowledge or say out loud to anyone. I had no idea how to express the agony I felt in my heart about people who died and relationships that ended poorly. I didn't know how to admit or even acknowledge to myself how much pain I was experiencing, let alone to anyone else. Vulnerability was terrifying, and, like many of us, hiding and pretending were the safer routes to take.

So I hid in my relationships. I hid my coping mechanisms. I hid the hurts and the habits I felt ashamed of. I pretended everything was okay—sometimes even to myself! Plastering a big smile on my face at church, sweeping issues under the rug at home, ignoring my tendency to take on too much responsibility at work. I performed for my extended family, hoping they wouldn't notice the things I tried to cover up. I felt scared all the time. Scared to show myself. Scared to be myself. Scared to tell the truth about my pain. The last thing I felt in my relationships was safe.

I remember a moment in counseling when the light bulb lit

up. My counselor said, "Irene, we create our own misery. *The battle starts in our minds.*" Our emotions and our bodies send signals to our brains that it's time to deal with something. The problem is that when we are unaware of or disconnected from the emotions or our bodies, we don't notice or listen to what the signals are trying to tell us to address. This impacts our behaviors both consciously and unconsciously. My behavior of medicating with alcohol was leading to my sense of isolation and powerlessness. But I was clueless about the fact that the negative cycles in my thought life and my emotional world were the source of my motivation to medicate in the first place.

Before there was a drink to anesthetize my pain as a child, there was a mindset to trap me into a negative way of thinking, which turned into a cycle of pain that cried out to be numbed. A mindset that led to negative self-talk, distorted thinking, blaming others, or denying my issues held me back. I struggled to define what was real and truthful versus what was a story or script I made up about something I experienced. These dysfunctional cycles began in my mind and compounded into debilitating emotional pain that would eventually lead to medicating and then my full-blown addiction.

Even as a child, I inherited ways of thinking and seeing the world that started me on the path of hiding, pretending, and performing. We all parent out of our experience of how we were parented, often unconsciously doing things because that is all we know. My mom did the best she could with what she knew at the time—spanking and yelling, which for my personality was more harmful than helpful as a form of discipline. I was desperate not to get in trouble. I did anything to avoid feeling shame or getting a spanking, which meant hiding, lying, and pretending much of the time.

Sharing about what happened in our family was looked down upon and had consequences. With the no-talk rule being the standard in our family, I was never able to learn to verbalize how these experiences growing up impacted me emotionally. Negative cycles can start from our dysfunctional upbringings or sometimes because of unacknowledged traumatic or stressful circumstances with our families of origin.

Even our families can be unsafe sometimes. We store information in our brains based on early experiences and naturally begin to anticipate our response. Our origin stories set the pace for our attachments and connections with others in adulthood, because our worldviews are through the lenses of the early messages we received from them. Negative early experiences become threats to our ability to bond in healthy ways as adults.

We *all* come from dysfunctional family systems. Perfect people, parents, and households don't exist. Every home has issues, dysfunction, problems, and pain that must be addressed and faced at various times. Now that I have my own family, I often tell my kids that I have no problem paying for their counseling visits well into adulthood! I recognize my dysfunctional impact on their upbringing. All parents are imperfect because we are imperfect human beings. Our past impacts our present. We behave today out of what we know from our past experiences all through childhood and into adulthood. Our experiences shape us into who we become as adults. When left unaddressed, our past leads to distress in our adult lives, as well as potential mental health issues, relational issues (with self and others), dependence issues, and overall developmental immaturity. But when it is addressed, the pain from our past can be healed.

Crazy making is a term used in the recovery world to describe how our minds become hijacked by our addictions and we make up

a false reality. We are no longer in control of the changes that happen in our
brains as a result of addiction. Our reasoning is off, and reality is distorted.
We create prisons of our own making,
and they start in our minds.

> We *all* come from dysfunc-
> tional family systems. Perfect
> people, parents, and house-
> holds don't exist.

I remember learning for the first time in rehab about the concept of being a functional adult. *What is a functional adult anyway?*
I thought to myself. Our facilitators taught us that functional adults
are those who are in touch with their inner worlds and their deepest
feelings. They have affirming relationships with themselves and
know how to honor and respect themselves. This allows them to
fully engage in relationship with others in a healthy way, trusting
their intuition and gut.

I always wondered why I had such deeply rooted self-esteem
issues growing up. The result of low self-esteem manifested in cycles
of self-defeating thinking, promiscuity, and behaviors that were not
serving me well. I had what I like to call "other-esteem" rather than
self-esteem. I cared more about what others thought of me than of
how I felt about myself! I made decisions largely out of the motivation of what others would think or how they would feel about
a decision, rather than honoring myself and how it impacted me.
These were all symptoms of the underlying issue of codependency
I did not yet recognize or understand.

Codependency is defined in several ways, but the clinical definition says that at the most basic level it is a psychological condition
in which persons feel an extreme dependence on certain loved ones
in their lives.[1] Pia Mellody, a nationally recognized authority on
codependence, refers to codependence as a disease and says, "Because
of dysfunctional childhood experiences a codependent adult lacks

the ability to be a mature person capable of living a meaningful life. Two key areas of a person's life reflect codependence: the relationship with the self and relationships with others."[2] Mellody teaches that codependents have difficulty experiencing appropriate levels of self-esteem, setting functional boundaries, owning and expressing their own reality, taking care of their adult needs and wants, and experiencing and expressing their reality moderately.

I was clueless about the impact of codependency on my development into adulthood, my thinking, and my emotional reasoning. Without understanding why we do what we do and recognizing the poor patterns of relating we inherited from our childhood, we remain helpless to change. But be encouraged. The Holy Spirit helps us in our weaknesses (Romans 8:26), and as we heal and grow in God and through relationships with healthy people, we find the capacity to change. (I will talk more about codependency, what it is, and how to cope with and recover from it in chapter 8.)

Safe People

No wonder we are terrified to change or to share! It is people who have hurt us the most in this world, yet it is people who will help us heal. Honestly, until the light-bulb moment with my counselor, I was almost certain that *other people* were creating my misery, not me! The journey to safety includes others. I wish we could go off to an island somewhere, solve all our problems, and come back ready to live our lives. Wouldn't that be nice? But as it turns out, we need others and others need us. This is no accident. God created us to be interdependent on one another, and we experience the fullness of His goodness and grace through others. Our brokenness is not something to be ashamed of; it is something to share with others for the purpose of healing, restoration, and redemption.

But how do we know whom to trust? How do we become trustworthy for others ourselves, so that we all can combat shame and isolation? So that we can resist feeling the compulsion to hide, pretend, and perform, in order to be accepted and loved? First, we must learn how to identify safe people.

Safe people are honest and humble and able to admit weaknesses. They confess failures and make amends. They are self-aware and use assertive communication, speaking the truth with kindness and candor. They maintain a mindset geared toward growth. Safe people do not gossip about others, mock them, or tear them down. They make us feel "at home" in ourselves, safe to be who we are. Healthy people confront others in a life-giving way and invite them to grow and change.

In their bestselling book *Safe People*, Dr. Henry Cloud and Dr. John Townsend define safe people as those who "draw us closer to God, to others, and help us become the real person we were created to be."[3] Why do we struggle to be this kind of person and to identify safe people as well? Likely because we have experienced quite the opposite in *unsafe* people. Perhaps you are like me and have been betrayed, judged, bullied, or talked about by unsafe people. Or maybe you have been unsafe and gossiped and judged other people—if we are honest, all of us have at some point in our lives—and you believe this is normal or acceptable behavior. You can spot an unsafe person if you notice they are easily triggered, can't get over their past, blame others, and have a hard time forgiving others or acknowledging when they make mistakes. They are repeat boundary violators and do not honor when you set limits. If you have been violated by someone physically, verbally, or emotionally, especially by a family member or someone who was meant to protect you and love you, not harm you, then people may equal danger in your mind. You may view people through the lens of mistrust if you were hurt by a person in a place of power in your life like a boss, teacher, pastor, or coach who overtly or covertly harmed you. These experiences with unsafe people can lead us to believe the lie that we cannot trust people.

Toxic Shame and the Hijacked Brain

Did you know that shame and addiction can become *toxic* to our brains? The brain is one of the organs in our body that determines our basic functioning and flourishing. Our brains get hijacked by addiction when we go from liking something to wanting it and then craving it incessantly. Dopamine acts as a neurotransmitter in the brain, sending signals or chemical messages that activate the brain's reward system. The dopamine overflow gives the feeling of being high.[4] As we consume or misuse substances, like drugs or alcohol, for temporary dopamine release and a high, our reward system is triggered for pleasure, and we crave more of that "good" feeling. The problem with abuse of these substances is that it lowers our natural production of dopamine so that we have emotional lows when sober, and therefore we chase the high we had when using the substance. Our brains become hijacked by addiction when the reward system circuit is overloaded by abuse of a substance, and we no longer are in control of our desires and motivations for the substance. We now crave it and feel we need it to survive or to be happy, yet the crazy behaviors and guilt and remorse after using it contribute to further emotional lows, which lead to more craving to feel better, and we end up in a vicious cycle. We keep doing the same harmful thing over and over despite getting the same negative results. That is the definition of insanity.[5] The biological purpose of dopamine is to motivate life-sustaining behaviors, such as eating when hungry, by giving us pleasure when we do them. But the misuse of mood-altering drugs artificially creates this effect in a more efficient and intense way than through natural methods.[6]

Brené Brown, whom I will reference many times in this book because she is a shame researcher and a notable resource on the topic, said in her TED Talk *Listening to Shame*, "How many of you, if you did something that was hurtful to me, would be willing to say, 'I'm sorry. I made a mistake'? How many of you would be willing to say that? Guilt: I'm sorry. I made a mistake. Shame: I'm sorry. I am a mistake."[7] That was one of the lies living rent-free in my head for years: *God made a mistake when He created me.* I didn't understand the shame embedded in the foundation of who I'd become. It was debilitating and distressing. Guilt says, "I *did* something bad." It is meant to signal us to modify a bad, offensive, or out-of-moderation behavior that has negatively impacted ourselves or someone around us. It can help us make amends or apologize. Shame, on the other hand, says, "I *am* something bad." It hinders our connection with others and presses us deeper into hiding, pretending, and performing. We enter survival mode, which is often accompanied by coping mechanisms that hurt us rather than help us.

The late Dr. John Bradshaw, in his book *Healing the Shame That Binds You*, wrote about toxic shame being a disease and an emotional illness that causes complex inner disturbance, such as anxiety, depression, self-doubt, isolation, perfectionism, inferiority complex, feelings of inadequacy, and many other compulsive disorders.[8] Many become exhausted with chronic anxiety as they try to achieve a false sense of perfection. This was my story as well as the story of many other people who are unaware of the effects of shame on the brain, on our development into adulthood, and on our emotional responses.

Simply put, the brain stores our experiences in our awareness or consciousness so that we respond emotionally from this place. So when toxic shame has hijacked the brain and we are triggered by the emotion of shame, we automatically go into fight, flight, or freeze. When faced with shame, the brain reacts as if we are facing physical danger and activates the sympathetic nervous system, generating the protective response.

The flight response triggers the feeling of needing to disappear, and children who have this response will try to become invisible. This was my response. In comparison, the fight response expresses itself as verbal and behavioral aggression by the embarrassed person toward the one who caused them to feel ashamed. The freeze response is what normally occurs when people are facing trauma in which they feel trapped and powerless. The freeze response is what allows us to survive situations where intolerable things are happening to us. All have negative consequences, because these responses upset our ability to think clearly, which results in beliefs that we are stuck in a situation where we have no power because something is wrong with us.[9]

When we believe the lie that what happened to us is our fault, we become the victim, and the negative cycle in the mind perpetuates the toxic shame responses. I was unaware that I was stuck in the fight/flight/freeze response most of my childhood and well into my adult life.

Between alcohol and shame, my body was deteriorating quickly.

So were my relationships. Shame told me that no one could ever find out my secrets because they (or worse, I) would ruin everything. So I hid more and more and got deeper and deeper into my misery. In the last two years of my drinking career, my brain was mush. I no longer took interest in things that used to excite me, like reading a book or watching my son play soccer. Reading is difficult when you are tipsy and incoherent. I found myself reading the same paragraph over and over and eventually gave up. And I was miserable with hangovers at soccer games. *How could this happen to me?* I thought constantly. *I am a pastor. I am a mother and a wife.*

As addiction took over my life, as well as shame about my abuse of alcohol, suicidal thoughts increased. I even entertained thoughts of how my family and community would be better off without me. Maybe if something happened to me, I'd never have to tell people how bad things were. Think about that—I was so afraid of being vulnerable and telling the truth that I considered ending my life as an alternative. Have you been there? Are you there now? There is healing. There is hope.[10]

Our hearts, minds, and bodies work together to keep us healthy and strong. When we are dealing with fear or toxic shame, wrestling with addiction, or avoiding pain, it is easy to divorce ourselves from the physiological indicators that something is wrong and needs to be addressed. We feel emotions in our body. Shame is typically felt in our face, neck, and upper chest. It usually feels warm, like heat across the upper body. Some of us even get red. Guilt is felt in the gut and feels like a gnawing sensation. These bodily responses help us acknowledge what's happening in our head, heart, and gut. Best-case scenario, after acknowledging the emotion, these responses lead us to change our behavior. Then we can make things right with those around us whom we impact. However, in an unhealthy guilt and shame cycle, when we believe we are inherently bad, that something is wrong with us, we run from the indicators rather than embracing our humanity. The longer we run, the more we create road maps in our brains that undergird the return to the behaviors that are unhelpful, even harmful.

Shame was changing my brain chemistry, causing depression and more self-hate. Hoping to fix what I thought was just depression and anxiety, I visited a doctor in 2014, who prescribed depression medication. I did not share the truth about how much I drank when the doctor asked me how often I drank. I continued to hide my secret in shame. At this point, I had no idea how connected shame and drinking were to these symptoms. Besides, I figured if I could find something medically wrong with me, then Jimmy would be satisfied and understand better that I couldn't help the anxiety I was dealing with. Or even better, maybe if I controlled the anxiety, I wouldn't feel like I had to drink so much to make the anxiety go away.

The warning labels on the prescriptions the doctor gave me said I should not mix the medication with alcohol, which I chose to ignore. I continued to hide and abuse alcohol in secret. The monster of shame and dependency on alcohol was growing, and I couldn't stop it. Denial of my problem with alcohol allowed me to remain blind to the toxic shame living in me like a growing cancer. Acknowledging my inability to stop drinking would confirm what I feared: I wasn't just doing something bad; *I was bad*. The agonizing internal tension of being a good person while also being an alcoholic ate me up inside. I falsely believed that good people don't have problems, and they certainly don't have addictions.

The False Expectation for Perfection

Friend, where do we get this idea that we are supposed to be perfect; that we must never make mistakes; that we're not supposed to struggle with the complexities of our lives? What and who taught us that to be loved, we cannot be broken? The truth is, we're all broken. This is what it means to be human—we are not alone in our struggles, and the enemy of our souls does not want us to understand that the common ground we all share is our brokenness, our need for a Savior to help us, heal us, and connect us to Him and to each other.

Shame is not exclusive to people in addiction. All humans feel shame because all people make mistakes. But toxic shame threatens our core identity as human beings. We see this from the very beginning of humanity, in the book of Genesis. Adam and Eve made a mistake. They hid from God because they were ashamed. Instead of coming to God with what they'd done, they internalized their shame and hid, covered, and pretended like God couldn't see what they'd done. We assume that our worthiness before God has to do with our behavior and what we do for God, so we hide, pretend, and perform even for God! Just like Adam and Eve, we assume that if we make a mistake—or that when we make a mistake—we will lose relationship and suffer rejection or abandonment. Sometimes the mistake is so large that this is the case. For example, an extramarital affair may result in the loss of a marriage, or flying off the handle in anger may sever communication with our children or spouse. A severe betrayal may result in new boundaries or disconnection from a relationship. But overall, our mistakes do not have to end our relationships if we acknowledge them and make amends. We must stop expecting perfection from ourselves and from others.

That is unrealistic and hinders the possibility for vulnerability and reciprocity.

Our natural human response is to avoid pain, so when we experience the emotion of shame, we try to subdue it or mask it through perfectionism. Shame causes us to hide and pretend everything is okay in the attempt to protect ourselves from people looking down on us. Shame tells us not to acknowledge the reality of our shortcomings and imperfections. Shame lies and says we don't have what it takes to face our lives.

In my shame, I chose to live in denial and believe that I was in control of my consumption of alcohol. I continued to drink alone and hide, refusing to admit what was right in front of me. I abused alcohol. It didn't occur to me that it was not normal or okay for a grown woman to hide her drinking. A friend of mine says, "Whenever you're hiding something, you're hurting someone." Hiding hurt the people I love. Pretending caused toxic and unbearable shame. Performing created a sense of striving and avoidance instead of peace and connection in my relationships with God, myself, and others. The need to be perfect separated me from others and increased my sense of aloneness.

Here's something I didn't fully understand at the height of my addiction: I was an emotional infant in my midthirties. I didn't have the emotional capacity to handle the weight and responsibility of overall life stress, full-time ministry, family, and marriage. I struggled to communicate and connect with others in an honest, healthy way. I struggled to confront others and deal with conflict and tension in a beneficial way and failed to realize that emotional health is directly connected to spiritual health. Emotional and spiritual health go hand in hand. The Bible is chock-full of examples of how our emotional world impacts our spiritual world. Science is finally catching up to Scripture. In chapter 8 we will dive deeper into the importance of emotional health in recovery.

The 12-step program adopted by Alcoholics Anonymous simply walks out principles that line up with the Bible, such as admitting our issues (sins) and confessing them to God and others. The steps involve recognizing the reality that our spiritual world and emotional world work hand in hand to aid us in overcoming addiction and coping differently with stress. Perhaps if we take a moment to read the 12 steps of recovery programs, we can begin to understand how they can apply to all of us and how beneficial they can be to our overall growth and health.

Here are the 12 steps defined by Alcoholics Anonymous that can be applied to any area of recovery we may be in:

1. We admitted we were powerless over alcohol—that our lives had become unmanageable.
2. Came to believe that a Power greater than ourselves could restore us to sanity.
3. Made a decision to turn our will and our lives over to the care of God as we understood Him.
4. Made a searching and fearless moral inventory of ourselves.
5. Admitted to God, to ourselves, and to another human being the exact nature of our wrongs.
6. Were entirely ready to have God remove all these defects of character.
7. Humbly asked Him to remove our shortcomings.
8. Made a list of persons we had harmed and became willing to make amends to them all.

9. Made direct amends to such people wherever possible, except when to do so would injure them or others.

10. Continued to take personal inventory and when we were wrong, promptly admitted it.

11. Sought through prayer and meditation to improve our conscious contact with God, as we understood Him, praying only for knowledge of His will for us and the power to carry that out.

12. Having had a spiritual awakening as the result of these Steps, we tried to carry this message to alcoholics, and to practice these principles in all our affairs.[11]

The 12-step program causes us to address our issues with unforgiveness and resentment and forces us to look honestly at our dysfunctional attitudes and behaviors in how we relate to ourselves, others, and God. These patterns of dysfunctional relationship with ourselves and others are what lead us to the abuse of a substance or drug of choice. The thought is, if we work on these areas consistently, we can change our inner world by learning to deal with our issues rather than medicating them with self-defeating coping mechanisms. The Celebrate Recovery program is a Christ-centered recovery program that expounds on the application of these principles to our lives in any area we need recovery in, whether a hurt resulting from trauma, a hang-up like unforgiveness, or any habit that has become an addiction.[12]

Addictions fall into two main categories, both of which start with deep chemical changes in the brain. *Substance addictions* involve chemicals. Common examples are alcohol, caffeine, marijuana, nicotine, cocaine, heroin, and prescription medications, including barbiturates, which are in many anxiety or sleeping medications. *Process addictions* involve our behavior. Common process addictions include gambling, pornography, shopping, gaming, workaholism, exercise, codependency, and love addiction.

Our brain cells are designed to respond to triggers that make us feel happy, like when a baby laughs or we smell food we love. With addiction, the same wonderful trigger gets set off in our brains when we use a substance or take part in certain activities. The spike of these happy feelings makes us want more. Over time the overuse of the addictive substance or behavior begins to escalate and make a mess of the pleasure cells in our brains, and they don't work correctly. Now we feel a compulsion to experience and chase that pleasure feeling, resulting in something harmless becoming harmful to us.

Do you see yourself—or perhaps a family member or loved one—in this type of situation? Throughout these pages I offer help for navigating your situation, providing practical tools for recovery and hope for healing. Because I was unaware of how addiction worked, it crept up on me without my knowing it. My parents were not heavy drinkers, and no one ever spoke about anyone in the family who were alcoholics or struggled with addiction, so it didn't occur to me that it could happen to me. I didn't will it on myself, but the pain felt too big to touch, and I was clueless about how to deal with it in a healthy way. The shame felt like part of my identity—I didn't know how to live without it. My coping mechanisms, even though they were negative, were meeting a legitimate need—illegitimately. I was ignorant of being ignorant, as Maya Angelou expressed in *I Know Why the Caged Bird Sings*. We only know what we know, so as a result of my ignorance of alcohol dependency, I unknowingly fell into the cycle of addiction through my continued heavy and frequent use of the substance.

We all have things we have yet to learn. Hopefully you will become more aware, and as you do, trust that God is on your side, and that I am here as a friend and a guide. I, just like you, may have been developmentally stunted as a child, but the good news is that we all can grow up anytime we choose. I grew up when I addressed my past. I grew up when I acknowledged the pain and traumatic things that happened to me as a little girl. I grew up when I faced the reality of who I was outside of what I did.

> My coping mechanisms, even though they were negative, were meeting a legitimate need—illegitimately.

At the tipping points of our lives, we have incredible opportunities to change the trajectory of our paths. Take some time for introspection, asking yourself if you are pretending to be someone you are not, and why. Who are you pretending to be? Are you performing for others and not honoring your deepest needs and wants? Are you hiding areas in your life? In what areas of your life is shame showing up? How is it preventing you from being your best self? Are you "using" something to numb or cope with your inner world being out of control? Is alcohol, food, or whatever you are using getting in the way of your life? Are you willing to face the shadows of your past that haven't been dealt with so you can be free from the baggage and weight of it? As James Baldwin said, "Not everything that is faced can be changed; but nothing can be changed until it is faced."[13] Crisis and pain can be the best teachers in life. Our greatest pain and misery have the potential to launch us into our greatest ministry, where we finally live out our purpose if we are willing to get honest, stop pretending, and do the work to break the cycles that threaten to take us out.

God accepts us as we are, on the way to where we are going.

He loves us as we are but loves us too much to leave us there. Have you heard that before? It's true. You are loved, just as you are, right where you are, flaws and all. And you can trust that God, in His loving-kindness, will not leave you in your pain, dysfunction, or addiction. You have what it takes to overcome, and when you don't, God does. And often He shows up through the people who love us the most.

CHAPTER 3

The Difficult Conversation You're Avoiding

*N*ovember 12, 2015, *was my last drink.* I was at the Baltimore/ Washington International Thurgood Marshall Airport. I'm glad I didn't know it at the time because I would have drunk myself into a sleepy oblivion. Like a greedy newborn puppy blindly and frantically searching for satiation from its hunger with its mama's breast milk, my eyes scoured the airport eating area looking for my next drink. *Aha!* The sushi place had individual bottles of chardonnay, so I purchased four. A sense of relief and urgency flooded me as I paid for the bottles, while glancing over my shoulder to ensure no one was looking. It wasn't even noon, and I was buying wine. I poured it into a cup, and presto!

I discreetly had my fix at the gate while waiting for my plane to Ohio. My friend Jennifer was anxiously awaiting my arrival in hopes of talking some sense into me. Jimmy was at his wit's end and gave me the ultimatum that if I did not get help and go to rehab, he was going to divorce me. I needed an intervention because his angry words were not driving me to change or get help but rather pushed me to dig deeper into my stubborn stance of defiance to do the opposite. Believe it or not, I still didn't think of myself as an alcoholic. Even with all the signs present, I continued to ignore them and function in complete denial of the reality of my dependence on alcohol.

I boarded, then tried to buy more alcohol on the plane, but the turbulence kept flight attendants from servicing passengers. Frustrated to no end, I will never forget the face of the woman sitting next to me as I complained bitterly that they weren't serving drinks. Then diarrhea of the drunken mouth ensued, and I was spilling my guts about how I didn't get why it was such a big deal for people to drink and why people judged those of us who wanted to drink. I was a blubbering mess, playing the victim, trying desperately to get someone to confirm that all my irrational thinking was true. She did not fall into my ploy to manipulate her into confirmation bias. In fact, she proceeded to tell me she had made a choice not to drink at all anymore and how it had changed her life for the better. *Weirdo. A life without alcohol? No way!* I thought to myself, silently judging her for her choice to abstain from alcohol. *I don't have a problem with alcohol, and if I do, it's my problem. I want to be left alone to it.*

Jennifer would later tell me that when I arrived in Cleveland, she could smell the wine on my breath, no matter how much gum I chewed to try to mask the scent of alcohol. She took me to Chipotle in hopes of feeding me so I could sober up. Mind you, all I could think about was the fact that they sold beer and wine in the

Chipotle in Ohio. *Wow! My hometown needs to get on board—what an incredible concept,* I thought.

Jennifer took me to her house and insisted I take a nap. With the hard conversation ahead, she knew that talking to me under the influence would not work. Panic and shame overwhelmed me as I entered her home. Would her kids know why I was there? More panic flooded my body as I realized there was no way for me to get alcohol while I was at her house.

Looking Back

Now I can see how God was with me all along the way. He sent me that angel on the plane. I can see now very clearly what I could not see then with my hijacked brain. She was probably "a friend of Bill," which is a term meaning she was in the AA recovery program. She calmed my anxiety with her kind, nonjudgmental words and reassurance about not needing alcohol to keep her calm or to have fun. I feel confident now that she could see all the signs of my alcohol problem yet dealt ever so gently with me. No shame. No judgment. She didn't beat me over the head with what I "shouldn't do." She shared her story and expressed how a life without alcohol had benefited her.

In hindsight, when I reflect on Jimmy's ultimatum, the gentle angelic woman next to me during turbulence, and Jennifer caring for me with such grace, I can see how God positioned me where I needed to be and sent His helpers so that I could get free from my addiction. He led me straight into the conversation I didn't know I needed—an intervention where I wearily agreed at last to get help.

As I sobered up in Ohio, I thought to myself, *How did I get in so deep? Maybe I am in too deep and should just keep digging, because it feels like there is no way out of this nightmare.* What does it take for us to change? You would think that hearing my precious, innocent children describe themselves cowering in fear when Jimmy and I fought would get the message through my head that I had a problem and needed to stop drinking. Insanity! But that is how addiction works. Many addicts hear the stories of harm their behavior causes loved ones and are still unable to stop. That was true for me. In fact, I dove deeper into self-hate, rationalizing my behavior and toxic shame. The stories I told myself about why I drank were lies that helped me excuse my dependency on alcohol. *It's Jimmy's fault that we argue! The stress of life is too much for me to handle! I work so hard—I deserve to take the edge off!* Blaming others for and refusing to deal with my problems and my pain blinded me from seeing the truth of my addiction and the impact on my children, marriage, and friends. I couldn't and wouldn't admit I had a problem.

The Conversations I Didn't Want to Have

Opportunities for growth and change line the road to recovery. Usually, a loved one will ask the right question or plead with us to get the help we need. But when we are thinking with addict brain, it is hard to listen during these conversations, much less respond in a way that fosters change. For example, on several occasions people asked if I was willing to give up or cut back on alcohol. My response was a simple no. Over the course of a year, none of my counselors or close family friends could convince me to give up alcohol. I would try to drink less, and I could stop for periods of time, but when I drank again, I was back to the same place in blackout city. Many people rationalize they don't have a problem, just like I did, because we convince ourselves that since we can stop for periods of time, it must mean we have it under control. We are deceiving ourselves.

Then there was the last straw with Jimmy.

"I can't take it anymore, Irene! You have got to get help! You have a problem!" Jimmy yelled. He could no longer contain his anger toward me and the deep-seated hate he felt for the craziness I was causing our family.

"How can you choose alcohol over me? Our children?" He begged me to stop drinking, and he explained to me that he couldn't and wouldn't allow my obsession with alcohol to run our lives anymore.

"If you do not go to rehab, it will be the end of our marriage." This broke me. Again, I thought, *How could he do this to me?* The crazy making in my mind had me believing he was the enemy.

I had no idea my trip to Ohio to talk to Jennifer about my next steps would radically change the trajectory of my life. Jennifer and her husband, Jim, were longtime friends whom Jimmy and I agreed would be our safe couple that we could share anything with. In the safety of my friend and her home, Jennifer asked me important questions. "How do you feel about the state of where your life and marriage is?" She listened intently. She cried with me when I described my inner turmoil and the pain I was experiencing.

She confronted my crazy making, irrational thoughts, false beliefs, and blame shifting lovingly, not in a harsh or angry way. She asked me open-ended questions to force me to say out loud how unmanageable things were in my life. Hearing her say back to me what I was expressing helped me let down my guard a bit. I did sound a bit crazy; I admit it!

I will never forget Jennifer saying, "I am concerned for your well-being and that of your family. Would you consider going to get help? Irene, think of yourself as being sick and needing to go to a doctor in order to get better. There is no shame in that. In fact, I believe it is the bravest thing you will ever do. Do you want to get better? Going to rehab is the biggest gift you could give yourself, your children, and your husband."

"Me, brave? I am a failure and a mess, Jen!" I struggled to wrap my mind around how rehab could be a *brave* thing rather than a shameful thing. This impacted my soul. The *bravest* thing I could ever do? Get help? The conversations we don't want to have will help us see things clearly. They help us reframe our shame. Give us permission to name our need. Make it okay—even brave—to get help.

As I sit and ponder what impacted me most in our conversations and created a turning point in my life, a few things stand out. Jennifer had empathy toward my pain. She reminded me of God's love for me and that God wanted to heal me. Jennifer specifically was the one who reminded me of God's promises of forgiveness. She said, "If you seek forgiveness from Jimmy, your family, and the kids, you will get forgiveness from them too. You made a commitment to God through your marriage vows. You can't give up on that now. Remember the days when you weren't drinking and how you felt Jimmy's and the kids' love for you? You can have that again. But if you choose not to get help, you stand to lose that."

Finally, she reminded me of how the treacherous arguing at home over my drinking had reached a tipping point, impacting our children deeply. My oldest daughter, Kayla, had described to Jennifer how fearful and unsafe she and her siblings felt when Jimmy and I fought and when she found me passed out on the bathroom floor while Jimmy was out of town. Kayla said that at one point she gathered her siblings together in her room and wrapped her arms around them, covering their ears with pillows so they couldn't hear the explosive details of our fights. *What? Me? Hurt my kids? This could not be happening, because how could I hurt the people I loved most?* Through this conversation I really didn't want to have, the truth was beginning to sink in: I needed help. It was right in front of me all along.

"So what are you willing to do? Stay the same and lose everything, or give up something you love [alcohol] for something you love more, your family?" Jennifer didn't speak after asking me that question, and the room was silent for what seemed like hours.

"Okay, fine. I will go to rehab. But I get to pick which one."

Don't get me wrong. Though I finally gave in and agreed to go to rehab, I still didn't trust the loved ones who were urging me to go. Emotionally, I was kicking and screaming all the way to the Meadows Treatment Center in Wickenburg, Arizona, where I decided to go. In fact, I even needed a chaperone. A friend of mine was with me, and I wouldn't drink with her around. I was quite sure that if she were not with me, I would have taken my drinks in first class like a champ. I met others at rehab who described the moment they decided to go to rehab as being the most dangerous time because they felt like they needed to drink as much as possible since their alcohol was about to be taken away. Many arrived with scars and bruises from their last binges without the slightest idea of how they were injured.

Why does it feel like we can't admit the reality that is so plain to everyone else?

We cry, feeling sorrow, but with no intention of changing. We rationalize and shift blame in an attempt to avoid facing reality, as if denial of the issue will make it go away. I remember being

_____
Why does it feel like we can't admit the reality that is so plain to everyone else?
_____

inconsolable when extreme feelings of shame, embarrassment, and hopelessness hit me, as Jennifer kept reminding me of the state of my family and the pain Kayla, Jaden, Maya, and Jimmy were suffering because of my behaviors, blackouts, and denial. The remorse was there, but my brain couldn't stop thinking about the possibility of losing my numbing agent. At the time, I still couldn't imagine my life without it. I was confronted with the question, *What am I willing to lose to keep my love affair with alcohol going?* Was I willing to lose my husband and possibly custody of my children if Jimmy left me? In my heart, I thought, *You might as well just kill me now because I am nothing and will have nothing if I lose them.* But the truth is, I didn't trust them. Until the Ohio trip that led to rehab, nothing was enough to make me change—because they were trying to keep me from my best friend. Alcohol.

The Addictive Cycle Is Subtle Until It's Urgent

The definition of disease is "any harmful deviation from the normal structural or functional state of an organism, generally associated with certain signs and symptoms and differing in nature from physical injury. A diseased organism commonly exhibits signs or symptoms indicative of its abnormal state."[1]

Whether alcoholism is a disease has been a matter of debate. I believe it is. Addiction is harmful and is a deviation from the original intent of how God designed our bodies to function. A variety of signs and symptoms indicate that addiction causes injury to a human being's bodily functions, ultimately altering them from being normal to abnormal. Certain signs indicate when something once manageable and done in moderation is developing into a bad habit. Then new signs signify that the bad habit is turning into an addiction.

I knew absolutely nothing about these signs. *Merriam-Webster* defines addiction as "a compulsive, chronic, physiological or psychological need for a habit-forming substance, behavior, or activity having harmful physical, psychological, or social effects and typically causing well-defined symptoms (such as anxiety, irritability, tremors, or nausea) upon withdrawal or abstinence."[2] In the clinical sense, addiction is defined as a chronic, relapsing disorder characterized by compulsive drug seeking, continued use despite harmful consequences, and long-lasting changes in the brain. It is considered both a complex brain disorder and a mental illness.[3]

You may be asking yourself, *If it's not an addiction, how can I make sure it doesn't become one?* You may observe a problematic behavior in yourself or a loved one, but it is not yet life devastating, so you are wondering if it is a big deal and even needs to be addressed. The addictive cycle is subtle until it's urgent, my friend. One minute you are drinking or using a substance, person, or thing for fun or relief, and the next thing you know it has developed into something you feel you need in order to survive and cope. For me, it was as if I added alcohol back to my life, and then I blinked, and suddenly I was faced with an ultimatum from my husband and had hit rock bottom. The consequences were urgent, and my response and decision to change my behaviors would ultimately determine the course of the rest of my life for the better or for the worse. Thank God I chose better and got help.

What Is the Spectrum? How Do I Know Where I Am on It?

Alcohol users fall into three main categories: social drinkers, alcohol abusers, and alcoholics. I was not aware of the different types of drinking patterns prior to getting treatment for my alcoholism. I wonder sometimes, if I had known, if I would have allowed myself to go so far down the scale. After all, alcohol is an addictive substance, so whether or not we are aware of the spectrum, we can easily travel down it.

For me, vacation was a great time to let my hair down and enjoy a drink prior to my slide down the slippery slope of alcohol addiction. I remember sitting by the pool relaxing and unwinding with a cold, deliciously refreshing mojito or margarita. Then it would be a cocktail before dinner, a few glasses of wine at dinner, then a nice dessert drink like a glass of caramel-flavored Bailey's Irish Cream over ice to finish off my night. Seemed harmless enough. Normal enough. Because everyone does it, right? That is, until I began ordering extra shots in my drink by the pool so that by the time I got to dinner I was already tipsy and headed toward a drunken stupor. I would say to myself, *This is only for vacation.* But once I got home, I wanted that great relaxing feeling to continue and would drink at the same "vacation" rate. I never stopped to think that at some point I needed to come back from vacation.

Can you relate to anything I have described? Do you find yourself rationalizing your use of a substance or behavior to address a legitimate need to relax or de-stress? If you got honest and examined yourself, might you see how you may be rationalizing your use, heading down a slippery slope as you begin to understand how addiction is a progressive disease? It's subtle. You may not even see it coming because it is hiding out in denial and lack of awareness.

This idea that there is a sliding spectrum to addiction can be applied to anything in our lives that we may use, whether it is a person, place, or thing. If we can understand the sliding spectrum of addiction, we can learn to identify when we are on a slippery slope toward addiction rather than engaging in a harmless habit. We don't have to hit rock bottom, because we can identify whether we need to get help before our lives become unmanageable.

From low risk to high risk and everything in between, there is not a one-size-fits-all treatment or response for how to deal with where we fall on the addiction spectrum. When we are considered low risk, we are not consuming or using at a harmful level. We should simply be aware that there is a potential for abuse if we are not moderating ourselves, especially if we have underlying factors like genetic or mental health issues that can play a part in how quickly we slide down the addiction slope.

Perhaps you noticed that when you went from working a forty-hour week to sixty hours and your body started breaking down and your relationships began failing—that is, negative consequences started increasing—that was the sign that you had crossed over from low-risk use of work for self-gratification to high-risk. Do you use work to make yourself feel better about your worth and value? Are you aware of when you are overworking so that you can make behavioral adjustments before you go down a slippery slope? Do you notice if your motivation to work shifts from providing for your needs to your enhancing your identity? Have you reached a point where, when you have lost relationships you neglected, you found yourself feeling hopeless, in shame, and rationalizing your choices, yet not able to slow your pace despite the toll it is taking on your health and relationships?

Just take a moment to consider where you fall on the spectrum. Where do you see yourself? Don't freak out and close this book and give up because you see yourself headed toward the high-risk portion of the spectrum. Honestly, the drinking Irene, who was in denial and running from her problem, would probably have done the same thing because I didn't want anyone to point out my alcohol problem. The shame that I had a problem made me want to deny it. I wanted to stay in my situation and be left alone. Just keep reading and allow awareness and your gut to direct you. When in doubt, talk to someone—a doctor or a friend—and do an assessment of yourself. No matter how far down the scale you have gone, there is a way forward, and your experiences can and will ultimately benefit yourself and others.

If your symptoms are indicating that you are beyond moderation in the use of a substance, person, or thing and you feel that you may be sliding down the addiction slope, a health professional can conduct a formal assessment to see where you stand. In the case of alcohol, a professional can assess whether alcohol use disorder is present.[4] Counselors are a great help in assessing our lives—not just substance abuse or use, but any other areas that are disrupting our lives or creating unmanageability.

Reframe, without the shame, the *name* of whatever is holding you back from getting help. What narrative or script can you reframe today? Here are a few ideas about how to change your perspective:

RECOVERY IS A BAD WORD AND DOESN'T APPLY TO ME. →
Recovery means I am healing.

GOING TO REHAB BRINGS UP SHAME IN ME. → I am being brave by getting help.

GETTING THERAPY MAKES ME WEAK. → Talking about my pain makes me strong.

I HAVE AN ADDICTION. → I have an understandable coping mechanism that I have taken to an extreme.

ATTENDING A 12-STEP PROGRAM IS EMBARRASSING. → Adopting weekly rhythms of support is the key to my breakthrough.

I NEED TO BE FIXED. → I have an opportunity to be brave.

WHAT IF I CAN'T DO THIS RECOVERY THING? → What if I *can* do this recovery thing?

Shame cannot survive when it is brought to the light. Shame cannot survive when we share our stories. In recovery, as we reframe the shame that is holding us back, we begin to see the world through new lenses. When we change our perspective, what we see changes.

I have learned in recovery to embrace pain and not avoid it. I have learned to kiss the wave though it made me seasick at times! Trials teach us hard lessons, and I hate to say it, but pain is a great teacher. Even better, though, is allowing *my* pain to be *your* teacher so you don't have to go through what I went through.

Second Corinthians 4:8–9 promises, "We are pressed on every side by troubles, but we are not crushed. We are perplexed, but not driven to despair. We are hunted down, but never abandoned by God. We get knocked down, but we are not destroyed" (NLT). Troubles will come from all directions, and we may feel helpless to control the outcome of our situations. But God promises that we will not be crushed or defeated by the enemy. Because God loves us, He will never abandon us. We don't have to despise the past or look back on it with regret. We can become thankful for our struggles and our crises, no matter how painful, because without them we never would have found our strength or experienced the grace and mercies of God in our lives.

Hurts, Habits, and Hang-Ups

A hurt, habit, or hang-up can derail us from God's original intent for our lives. If you are breathing and walking on this earth, you are likely dealing with a hurt right now. Every day internal and external habits are guiding your lifestyle and behavior. And potentially you have a hang-up in your life hindering you from flourishing. Let me explain these more clearly. A hurt is something painful we have experienced, such as a trauma. A habit is something we continue to do despite harmful consequences, for example, a substance or behavior/process addiction. A hang-up is anything we refuse to let go of that is not benefiting us in a positive way, such as unforgiveness, resentment, codependency, or family dysfunction. If you are unaware that you struggle with any of these, you are in danger of your life and relationships taking an unintended detour.

Denial of reality can cause us much harm. Consciously or unconsciously avoiding or even refusing to face and accept reality in our lives causes problems. Yet we do this as a protection mechanism to avoid feeling the pain of a situation or the reality that something painful happened in our lives. God said in Jeremiah 6:14: "You can't heal a wound by saying it's not there!" (TLB). We can't climb out of distorted or skewed ways of perceiving things or people until we give ourselves permission to admit that "it" happened or "it" was painful.

One of my hang-ups was that I became an expert at repressing my painful emotions from the hurts in my past and my present. This became an internal hang-up when I would evaluate my worth and value in this world, which manifested as the consequence of depression and anxiety. Undealt with pain will do that to us. When we don't deal with and release pain, we pick it up and carry it with us wherever we go. The pain, stress, and trauma come out somehow. We reach for something to cope, then repeat the painful pattern. Perhaps it's overeating or drinking, or lack of capacity for basic hygiene and self-care. Maybe it's through contentious relationships, procrastination on projects, or overachieving at work. It's only a matter of time before we break down as a result of undealt-with pain. Our bodies don't forget trauma and pain. We have to process trauma and pain for them to be released. Otherwise, they compound.

Our responsibilities in life are already heavy. Do you feel that way—so overwhelmed at times, you just want to pull the covers over your head and sleep for three days straight? When we add all the emotional baggage we pick up along the way in life and don't offload, eventually we will fall flat on our faces from the weight of it. I know about that. I carried a boatload of weight that I picked up throughout my childhood, with no idea how the heaviness impacted my present. With no tools to unload the weight, I felt broken and miserable, and I was unraveling. Alcohol helped me pretend that the flashbacks of childhood sexual abuse did not really happen. Denial protected me for a while. I thought denying the abuse would keep me safe. I drank at my pain to numb my emotions; however, I didn't anticipate all my emotions going numb, including the good ones like joy, peace, and happiness. When you attempt to numb one, you actually numb them all.

If we take a moment here for you to be really honest with yourself, is there an area of your life that has or is becoming unmanageable because you keep repeating a behavior that has harmful consequences? Is there a hurt you are ignoring? A habit you are hiding? A hang-up causing you to lose your peace?

Remember, no one can hear your thoughts—I don't know what you are afraid to admit to yourself, but my hope is that this will be a safe place to explore the things that are hindering you from living the life you dream of. I know it can feel absolutely terrifying. You wonder, *What will be on the other side of my acknowledgment that I have a hurt, hang-up, or habit? What will the people in my life think if they find out? What will I have to give up to be well?* Friend, I get you. The mere thought of admitting my issue sent me into a tailspin of denial. Not everyone in your life will understand how hard it is to admit that you have a problem and need help. But I promise you this: on the other side of denial is the beginning of freedom. Ephesians 4:25 says, "Stop lying to each other; tell the truth, for we are parts of each other and when we lie to each other we are hurting ourselves" (TLB).

We have to stop lying to ourselves. Get real with ourselves. Get honest—truly honest. I get that it is hard sometimes to do this. As you can already see from my story, the struggle to get honest was real. I didn't know how to do that. Denial was easier. In fact, I remember being in counseling with my husband and asking the counselor, "How does he do that? I mean, how does he just say what is on his mind? He is brutally honest." I said this as if honesty is a bad thing. Her response shook me to my core: "It's called being honest. You should try it sometime."

> I promise you this: on the other side of denial is the beginning of freedom.

This conversation with my counselor prior to rehab confronted my processing and caused me to consider reality. Would I continue to self-sabotage my own healing and happiness because of the inability to get real with my issues and my dysfunction? A breakthrough could happen if I began to be truly honest and stopped hiding the truth about me from myself.

PART 2

Accept

The Way Out

CHAPTER 4

Reframe Your Story

I don't remember my early days in Zambia, East Africa, where I was born, but I have heard stories of the beautiful property my parents owned, the twenty-five-acre farm with a home and guest quarters. My father was a professor at a teacher training college, and my mother was a teacher and a mother of five. We left Zambia abruptly to move to Connecticut, where my father was from, and my mother welcomed her sixth child to the world. I remember my mom telling me stories of how she grew up in Zambia. Imagining myself in her world, I'd picture her as a little girl skipping around her village, following behind her mother like a little duckling wherever she went. I loved hearing her stories! In our family, this tradition of storytelling ensured we understood and didn't forget the lives of those who went before us. Storytelling gives us insight into our history and heritage and acts as a way to preserve traditions and cultural knowledge from one generation to the next.

So much of our past plays a part in our present. When I checked

> Storytelling gives us insight into our history and heritage and acts as a way to preserve traditions and cultural knowledge from one generation to the next.

into rehab, one of the first exercises we had to do in counseling was create a timeline of major events that marked our lives from birth to present and shaped us in negative and/or positive ways. Acknowledging them was a task that took some time to muster up the courage to do, but true to my history of being a good student, I took on the homework assignment with the intention of completing it and getting the A+ of approval I wanted from my counselor. As a professional people pleaser new to recovery, I dove right in and tried to do my best to please my counselor with my work.

I remember being in group counseling, listening to others in my group share what they wrote on their life timelines. I began to hear all kinds of stories of childhood abuse, abandonment by parents, times when something impacted them in big ways, and how those experiences were still mysteriously active and alive in their present lives. For some, it was almost as if those difficult and traumatic events happened yesterday. People experienced physical manifestations of anxiety and depression, which led to attempted suicide, debilitating migraines, and mental torment; some led to addictions of all kinds.

The counselors diagnosed me with post-traumatic stress disorder (PTSD) stemming from a slew of traumatic events I had experienced in my childhood and on into adulthood. Hearing the others in my group share, I began to realize as I worked on my own list of life events that I had minimized big traumas (big T's) and altogether ignored little traumas (little t's) in my own life.[1]

I was learning that the big T's and little t's, whether we acknowledge them or not, shape us throughout the course of our lives into who we are as adults. And significant damage is caused in our development as children when these traumas go unaddressed, which had certainly been the case for me. Developmental fractures, stemming from things like abandonment and neglect, that force a child to figure out life on their own, cause us to grow into emotionally stunted adults with relational dependency issues. This can create crippling issues in adulthood behavior when a person becomes overly dependent on others for basic day-to-day life functions, or the complete opposite extreme, where they are needless/wantless and don't ask for help from others, don't know how to acknowledge when they need something, and don't even know that it is okay to take care of their wants in life.

I could relate to the latter extreme. I took care of myself in ways that should have had adult support or guidance. I never asked for help and didn't even realize I was allowed to have things I *wanted* because I was overly concerned with meeting the needs of others, while quietly resenting them for not taking care of themselves and their own needs and wants. Let me break this down for you: If I was tired, I felt guilty resting. I had a hard time spending money on myself or treating myself to something, taking on the mentality that I wasn't worthy of nice things. I had unconsciously picked up many of my behaviors from my parents through the filters of a child's mind, which became my experience, my truth, the way I functioned as an adult. Do you know that just because you experienced something as normal in your childhood does not make it healthy or right?

A child's experience compared to an adult's is very different. Children cannot be expected to process something the way an adult does, because their brains are not developed cognitively. Yet we sometimes expect them to react, respond, or process as an adult would. According to neurologists, the human brain isn't considered "adult" or fully formed until age twenty-five or twenty-six.[2] Executive functions, such as planning, working memory, impulse control, and judgment for decision-making, are slower to develop prior to the midtwenties. The prefrontal cortex is where our memory and information are stored and is developed through life experience, challenges, and other stimuli that can serve as a catalyst to "mature" some adolescents faster than others. Understanding and coping with big *T*'s and little *t*'s is difficult for children, teens, and young adults. Without support, therapy, or even language to describe and process pain, unhelpful and harmful habits and mindsets begin that lay the foundation for coping with life in adulthood.

For me, boarding school at age fourteen in Leysin, Switzerland, is where I had to figure a lot of life out on my own. I had been living abroad in Bamako, Mali, West Africa, for my eighth-grade year of school and was sent to boarding school for ninth grade. My father's job paid for students to attend boarding school because the American school in Bamako, Mali, only went through eighth grade.

Going to boarding school was an experience both my parents had at the age of fourteen, so it made sense to them for me to do the same. I had plenty of experiences to challenge me to mature quickly, as I had to figure out how to navigate the intricacies of typical adolescent challenges, such as friendship and the drama that went along with that, emotional crises, and self-esteem issues. I also entered puberty as a late bloomer and had to figure that out alone, along with managing the teenage embarrassment of things like acne breakouts, pain of menstrual cramps, and hormones that I didn't understand and made me feel out of control at times. I had no idea what to do. Thank God, my sister was in college in the United States, and I was able to call her sometimes for life instructions.

Prior to Mali and boarding school in Switzerland, I lived in the US, where I attended a portion of sixth grade and all of seventh grade. Prior to that, I lived in Cameroon, West Africa, where I was homeschooled after a failed attempt to attend a local Cameroonian school. Corporal punishment was a regular part of the school's disciplinary measures. I was terrified out of my mind to go to school (definitely a big *T*) for fear of being punished by the teachers. After my faking headaches for several weeks, and the school passing a rule that all girls had to shave their heads to avoid the spread of lice, my parents took us out of that school and hired a teacher to homeschool my brothers and me. The idea of shaving my head and the fear of being whipped with whatever instrument the teacher could find, like I saw happening to other children, was enough to cause a big *T* in any youngster. Witnessing trauma can sometimes be just as damaging to a person as experiencing it.

Prior to Cameroon, I had moved around Maryland with family, attending different schools. By the time I reached my senior year of high school, I had been at twelve different schools in all. Yeah, that is definitely an experience that shaped me—I had been the new girl twelve times and had no self-esteem and no emotional coping skills. All the moves created a series of little *t*'s that compounded into one big *T.*

Perhaps as you read my story, memories are stirred within you. We all have experiences that are little *t*'s and big *T*'s; however, we also carry memories of joy and peace in our relationships, of dreams and desires fulfilled. This is certainly true of my childhood. Alongside the scary, isolating lows on my timeline in rehab, I wrote down the positive moments that made me who I am as an adult. I was fortunate to have the opportunity my parents gave me both to go to school and live abroad. In Africa I got to see the "big five" animals on incredible family vacations and to meet and connect with people from all over the world. Living in the Swiss Alps, I skied to my heart's content and toured Europe as a freshman in high school, as well as Egypt for two weeks, where I saw the Great Sphinx of Giza and the pyramids with my very own eyes. The things I studied in history books, I also visited up close, and for that I am forever grateful.

So how did that young girl, with so much potential, education, and world experience, end up in rehab at age thirty-eight? How did I end up praying for the ground beneath me to swallow me whole because the pit of despair, shame, and hopelessness was too much to bear? Maybe you're there right now, reading these words and feeling seen, wondering how in the world you got where you are. Perhaps you are struggling emotionally and can't put your finger on the "why." The signs are there that your life is becoming unmanageable, maybe not from addiction, but you notice you can't handle things that you used to excel at, and you are baffled by that. Your employer is wondering what is going on with you because your work performance is diminishing to the point where your absentmindedness, mistakes, or lack of motivation can no longer be ignored. Maybe you have been put on performance improvement plans and have even been written up for your performance issues, but you don't see what your boss's problem with you is because you view the discipline as a personal attack rather than a growth opportunity. You could be silently saying to yourself (like I did all the time), *There is no way this can be happening to me! What is wrong with me!* Whether you are reading from rehab, suffering silently in your marriage or faith community, or feeling like there is no way out of the anxiety and exhaustion, I want you to know that you are not alone. Help is available. Your life is not over. I have been there, right where you are. There is a way out.

Choosing to get into treatment is not easy, and my friend Jennifer had her work cut out for her as we sat at her kitchen table in her home and scoured the internet together for a suitable treatment center that I was comfortable with. Anything close to my home was appealing because I would be close to my family; however, the thought of seeing someone I knew in treatment terrified me. I didn't want anyone to know or find out my shameful story. The Meadows Treatment Center was in Wickenburg, Arizona, and it was far enough away from people I knew and had the dual diagnosis approach to treatment that I needed. With hands trembling, I picked up the phone and punched in the number to speak to an intake specialist.

I cried incessantly on the phone with the intake specialist at the Meadows and asked questions about what my experience would be like. I also answered the questions she asked me. How much was I drinking? Was I having blackouts? Did I drink and drive? How were my relationships with family? The proof was in the pudding, so to speak. The realization was hitting me that I was in trouble and needed help fast.

After reluctantly agreeing to go to rehab, I had to fly back to Maryland to pack and say my goodbyes before leaving the next day. The intake specialist said I had forty-eight hours from the time we spoke to check in. I felt rushed and pushed in the moment, but I now understand the need to get someone into treatment as quickly as possible before they have an opportunity to change their mind.

The mere thought of saying goodbye to my family was turning my stomach upside down. Would leaving my children for forty-five days cause trauma for them? The script in my mind was saying, *You are a bad mother for leaving them*, and I believed it. Shame overwhelmed me. I still went to church that Sunday, shame written all over my face as I wept during praise and worship alongside my children. Jimmy stood next to me, with slight tears in his eyes from deep anger and pain. I remember the worship leader singing a song that encouraged me when I couldn't and didn't know how to pray. A war was going on in the spirit realm for my soul, and God was giving me supernatural confidence to trust that He would not allow death or addiction or trauma or fear or shame to win my soul. I belong to God. You do too. We are made in His image. He loves us. And friend, He holds you now, helping you all the way through. He is trustworthy and true.

James 4:7–10 says this:

> So let God work his will in you. Yell a loud *no* to the Devil and watch him make himself scarce. Say a quiet *yes* to God and he'll be there in no time. Quit dabbling in sin. Purify your inner life. Quit playing the field. Hit bottom, and cry your eyes out. The fun and games are over. Get serious, really serious. Get down on your knees before the Master; it's the only way you'll get on your feet. (MSG)

Finally, I'd hit rock bottom, crying my eyes out. The fun and games were over. Alcohol was no longer relaxing and enjoyable; it was evil and destroying my soul. All the lying, pretending, and avoiding big *T*'s and little *t*'s was done. Even my little *t*'s were compounding into a big *T*, and I was unraveling. Rehab was my quiet yes to God. I had no other choice but to trust that He would be there in no time, helping me get back on my feet again.

The Power of Storytelling

It was that small circle of people sharing their stories in rehab that helped me admit my struggle with alcoholism and codependency. When we hear someone's story and can relate, we experience a sense of solidarity and belonging. Knowing we are not alone in our struggles becomes tangible when we can say, "Me too!" It's interesting that the word *testimony* in Hebrew means "do again,"[3] signifying that what God did in one person's life, He wants to do again in ours. This gives us tremendous hope that we are not alone. Your sin is not special. It can be forgiven and healed, and you can be set free and redeemed, just like all the other folks Jesus loves. It's time for us to stop believing the lie that some sin is too hard for God, that it's too impossible to overcome. As the prophet Jeremiah wrote, "I am the LORD, the God of all the peoples of the world. Is anything too hard for me?" (Jeremiah 32:27 NLT).

Hope began to rise up in me—hope for freedom from addiction, restoration of my body and mind, transformation in my relationships with family, friends, and my faith community. I identified and related with many of the experiences and struggles I heard. These people were not broken-down drunks or defeated addicts with mental health issues. They were brave overcomers, courageous enough to get vulnerable and share their brokenness and experiences so we could find our breakthrough together! I benefited from their stories being shared just as much if not more than they did themselves. They were people from all walks of life—doctors, lawyers, stay-at-home mothers, nurses, grandparents, and young parents. From the outside, their lives would have looked normal, just like mine. Society tends to view addiction in such a negative light that we assume a caricature of a person struggles with this.

The truth is, anyone who lacks the tools, support, or willingness to examine why they do what they do is vulnerable to hurtful and harmful coping mechanisms, including addiction.

But their stories, varied as they were, inspired me to face my own story and move from avoiding the problem to admitting the problem. In that safe space, I discovered that I did not have to run from the past, hide from the past, or pretend to be perfect in order to be loved. I did not have to walk on eggshells around myself or my thought life. It was time to embrace garbage and dig up the dysfunction. I was ready, my brain was ready, and the sign I missed was hidden in what I saw as a midlife crisis. What I thought was a crisis was simply my brain saying it was time to deal, which is why memories were rising up. Our bodies tell us so much about what we can handle when we listen closely and get in touch with what we are feeling and what is coming up in our memories. If you are unraveling emotionally, I want to encourage you that you will not die, and you don't have to stay in your emotional crisis. You are at the incredible beginning of your breakthrough. Your crisis is not the end of you, nor is it your life sentence. It is the beautiful beginning of walking in freedom if you are willing to do the work to get free.

> The truth is, anyone who lacks the tools, support, or willingness to examine why they do what they do is vulnerable to hurtful and harmful coping mechanisms, including addiction.

Let me take a minute here to ask a few questions. Part of the reason I constantly asked, *How can this be happening to me?* is because I assumed I could never be one of "those people." So let's deal with that. How have you thought about addiction or about people with hurts, habits, and hang-ups? What are the judgments or assumptions you hold in your mind or heart about them? How did you develop these assumptions? Do they keep you from admitting your own struggles and character flaws? Why or why not? Sometimes pride can hinder us from getting the help we need. Allowing the Holy Spirit to help us view ourselves, the pain we (and others) experience, and our next steps for the future with humility and grace is key to sobriety and sanity.

It hit me like a ton of bricks on the evening of day 38, as I sat in yet another AA meeting where I continued to fight the notion that I was an alcoholic. The thought for the day was to look back over our drinking careers and consider how our lives were a mess because we were a mess inside.

Suddenly, through the power of a story, the fragmented pieces of my life began to click into place. All those years, it felt like I was looking at things through the bottom of a glass. My perception of reality was distorted the way the bottom of a glass distorts our vision, so that I couldn't see what was right in front of me clearly. I couldn't see the love of the people closest to me—my husband, children, friends, and family, and the God who loves me despite my craziness and brokenness. That's when I began to break free from the clutches of denial, slowly beginning to understand that I am loved and wanted, cared for and accepted.

The light bulb went on for me in a moment when the group was asked if perhaps their view of life was distorted because of looking at it through the bottom of a glass. When we look through the bottom of a glass, we can't see what is right in front of us. It is distorted. Our loved ones are right in front of us, but we haven't seen them. God has been with us all along the way, through ups and downs, bad choices, and consequences, and yet we still couldn't see Him in it all.

I began to consider that there wasn't a problem with life itself.

There wasn't a problem with God or with my family loving me. Life was good enough, but I was looking at it all wrong. I was looking at my life through the bottom of a wine glass, which was distorting my vision and perspective. I couldn't see clearly what was right in front of me—my family who loved me. My loved ones could see me, but I could not see them because my vision was blurry. I couldn't see the God who loved me or the husband who believed in me and wanted the best for my life. I couldn't see forgiveness from God and those I had hurt, which was mine to be had if I asked for it. Because of my distorted filter, I couldn't see all the beauty and purpose life had to offer me. I was blind, but suddenly I could see in that moment. The group leader asked this question: "Can you now look at life as it really is?" My palms began to sweat, and I became fidgety in my seat as the burning desire to raise my hand was forcing me to do just that. I felt that if I didn't raise my hand, I might explode on the inside.

Don't think. Just do it. Just admit it, Irene! Conquer the fear to admit it! This is your choice, I said to myself. *No one is forcing you, and you know too much now about how you got here. Just admit it!* I slowly raised my hand and made my first public admission of my alcoholism. "My name is Irene, and I believe I am an alcoholic." *Boom! There! I said it!* To my surprise, the room erupted in a resounding round of applause and cheers from my peers. I began to share how I related with all the stories. I had examined myself and could no longer deny my problem with alcohol. I shared about my session with my psychiatrist and how his words shook me to my core. My life had become unmanageable, and it was time to face reality. Step 1 of AA was complete and in the books!

After the meeting, my peers gave me hugs, high fives, and affirmation. They offered sincere congratulations for taking the first step in overcoming denial. A pivotal moment I will never forget was when my friend Michael gave me his precious one-year sobriety gold coin. He said that he had to do something special to commemorate this significant moment in my life because it was a big deal that I finally came to admit my issue. Other friends chimed in and said, "It's about time!" They already knew I was an alcoholic and had been patiently waiting for me to realize it on my own. I asked them why they hadn't said anything sooner if they knew and it was that obvious. They graciously reminded me that the journey was mine and that I needed to come to that place on my own.

In that one moment on day 38 of rehab, my miracle happened. Clarity came to me in an instant. The apostle Paul wrote in 1 Corinthians 13:12, "We don't yet see things clearly. We're squinting in a fog, peering through a mist. But it won't be long until the weather clears and the sun shines bright! We'll see it all then, see it all as clearly as God sees us" (MSG). This promise manifested in an AA meeting. I faced my fear of shame that I had a problem with alcohol. It would be the first of many moments in which I would learn the benefits of surrender. God's grace came into that moment and gave me the strength to face the days to come when I would be confronted repeatedly with the shame of the mess I had created of my life. My life after fear began on day 38.

"I think I'm an alcoholic, as much as I don't want to admit it. And I think I may have a desire to stop drinking." The burden continued to lift every time I showed up for a meeting and made a decision to honor my body, listen to my pain, connect to others, and ask for help.

I was beginning to realize that I was one of "them." Yeah, me.

An alcoholic. Allergic to alcohol. One drink is too many, and one thousand are not enough.

I want to tell you something you may not know. Recovery is not a "one and done" situation. Even if you end the addictive behavior with a final decision, that does not mean all your problems will go away. We do not go from the pit to the mountaintop and stay there. Healing is a process and is different for everyone. Wholeness and restoration are a process, and it's messy at times. We have to be gentle with and kind to ourselves as we allow our brokenness to speak to the way ahead. Recovery takes time, and there will be bad days, but overall, recovery leads to the kind of self-love we deeply and desperately crave.

Knowing When and with Whom to Share Your Story

When I returned from rehab, I was gripped with shame. I didn't want anyone to know what I had been through and what I had put my family through. I couldn't look anyone in the eye, even though I worked my internal shame meter down through my forty days at rehab. The toxic shame that originally caused depression and suicidal ideations was now a level of shame that in my newly sober mind felt more manageable. The affirmations I had learned to will myself out of those negative thought cycles helped manage the threat of shame attacking my mind. I now understood the power of shame to keep me bound in a negative opinion of myself and God. It was easier to see how shame had silenced me, left me suffering alone, feeling distant from God and others. With my new tools, I could fight that sense of isolation and embarrassment every moment of every day. Slowly, slowly . . . one day at a time, one step at a time, one moment at a time, one trigger at a time, one thought at a time.

Repairing my connections with my husband and family was important, even in that vulnerable place, fresh out of the treatment center. Jimmy and I looked for encouragement in others, hoping to find people willing to talk about their struggles now that we were facing our own. Jimmy's anger began to dissipate as he gained hope and faith in my recovery. As I worked my thorough recovery plan at home, sharing my aha moments, he felt encouraged that my recovery was real and that restoration was possible for our family. Every time I shared my experience of what I had learned about my issues and how to overcome them, my family's hope grew. We started to see a way forward that involved healing and gave more hope than I thought possible that things could get better. We could be restored.

Jimmy had begun to empathize with my struggle with shame, trauma, and addiction as he learned more and more about what I was experiencing. This took a lot of courage from me, because I had to open up, get vulnerable, and take the risk that he might reject me when I shared ugly things I was dealing with inside me. The more vulnerable and transparent I got with him, the more I built trust with him.

Three months after I returned home, Jimmy happened upon a Facebook post of a pastor's wife in Florida who was celebrating several years of sobriety. He encouraged me to reach out to this woman for support. I took the chance, not knowing what I would say when she answered the phone. When I sheepishly shared that I had just come home from rehab, I sensed her immediate acceptance and loving embrace in her voice through the phone. It was as if she was right in front of me, giving me a big hug and telling me,

"Honey, everything is going to be okay! I am so proud of you!" She became my safe place and a person I looked up to who had been on the recovery journey for some time and was thriving. She challenged and encouraged me and held me accountable to my growth process, becoming my sponsor, of sorts. She embodied all the qualities a sponsor should have and encouraged me to work my program. Having a sponsor can sometimes be intimidating if you aren't aware of the importance of having one in recovery. A sponsor is simply someone who can hold you accountable to the goals you set for yourself and who can share their own experiences of strength and hope as you process the unknown. The onus is on the person in recovery, not the sponsor. Since support is critical to recovery, finding a safe person to confide in who has been there and done that and who can guide you as you own your recovery process is vital.

My new sponsor's support felt especially helpful as I agonized over publicly sharing my addiction to alcohol. She told me it was okay to hold things close for a while, that it was okay to wait to share when I felt ready—and not a moment sooner. The pressure I was putting on myself about how and when I was to share my story was self-inflicted torture. I agonized over people finding out my secret struggle. I felt pressure to share what I had been through, but the stories I told myself about how I would be rejected, judged, and shamed terrified me into silence. She reassured me that I was putting unnecessary pressure on myself to share now. Who said it had to be now? It's okay to honor yourself and work through the fear and shame before even thinking about sharing publicly. I released myself from all that pressure when she reminded me of how Mary, the mother of Jesus, after the angel told her she would become pregnant by the Holy Spirit and give birth to Jesus, kept things close to her heart until the timing was right to share. Scripture says she "kept all these things in her heart and thought about them often" (Luke 2:19 NLT).

The Bible is rich with stories of people who are dealing with the same things we are. I identified with the shame Mary must have felt as a teenager, pregnant, and not by the man to whom she was betrothed. I can imagine her fear and apprehension to share about the baby she carried. What would people say or assume about her? While her story is not mine, I felt that same kind of fear she must have felt—fear of what people would say or do. What would the church congregation think of me? Would they reject me? Would my family be shamed by the fact that their daughter, wife, sister, mother, aunt, daughter-in-law was a drunk?

I made the decision to keep my situation and process close to my heart and to think and write about it often in the safety of my home with my immediate family, with close friends, in counseling, and at AA for a season, where I could keep my anonymity. God was working in me and developing credibility in my sobriety over time while I consistently worked at my recovery program every day for a little over two years. There's a quote I love, though the author is unknown, that says, "Work hard in silence and let your success make the noise." Deciding to grow in integrity and healing before inviting other voices and eyes into your life is wise. Critics and cynics are easier to handle when we know we are supported, surrounded, and loved, when we know that someone's words, disapproval, or actions will not have the power to take us on an emotional roller coaster, keeping us in turmoil.

Go slow. Protect your healing and recovery journey, especially when you are most vulnerable. Your greatest misery can become your greatest ministry, just like mine did. I will talk more in chapter 12 about turning your pain into purpose. But you must be wise in the timing of your sharing and with whom you share. Sharing in safe places at the right time is critical to the redemptive nature of your recovery journey. If you still feel acute shame, tears, and pain, I suggest working through things before you share them publicly. Your story may be meant just for one-on-one or small settings until you experience healing and breakthrough in whatever it is you are dealing with. To provide safety for yourself and others, establishing boundaries for sharing is imperative. If sharing a part of your story will hurt someone, you need to use discretion to protect their privacy (more on this later). Oversharing can be a boundary violation and instead hurt or trigger yourself or others. You must be mindful of this when sharing about abuse and naming individuals who have hurt you. Find safe places to share, like with a counselor or even in a journal, to process and keep your story close, working through your healing before you decide to share it more broadly, or even publicly. Not everything is meant to be shared publicly. Some things are for you and God to process. Some things may be shared with your spouse, a close friend, a teacher, a small group in your church, a recovery program, or a prayer partner.

Consider step 6 of AA: "Admitted to God, to ourselves, and to another human being the exact nature of our wrongs." Confession brings healing. When we confess our sins to God, we are forgiven (1 John 1:9), and when we confess our sins to others, we are healed (James 5:16)!

Freedom is on the other side of your sharing, which is why being part of a small group is so important. We learn in rows, but we grow in circles. Relationships and connection are basic human needs and bring us tremendous hope and healing.

Don't be ashamed of your story; it may inspire others! God is the author and the finisher of our faith *and* our stories, and He is not done writing yours. Will you let Him redeem and rewrite your story? All He needs is your willingness to be brave and share as He leads you.

CHAPTER 5

Reframe Your Recovery

The word *recovery* gets a bad rap. You may think recovery doesn't apply to you and it's just for "those people." I used to believe that people in programs like AA or Celebrate Recovery were not like me. Too often we think they have bigger issues than we do, and we reject the idea that we are like them. I felt the same way for a long time and was unaware of the purpose and content of those programs and their meetings. But when I began to dig deeper into my journey of recovery, I realized *recovery* is not a bad word. Turns out those groups are quite remarkable. Their tried-and-true practices produce joy and right living that compelled me to learn more because I wanted those things for myself. It's been said that "recovery is not for people who need it; it's for people who want it." We must reframe the shame of recovery if we truly want to get free from things that hold us back from being our best selves and living our best lives. Why have we been ashamed to pursue the rituals and weekly connections that can increase our joy?

The word *recovery* is defined as a return to a natural state of health, mind, and strength. It's the action or process of regaining possession or control of something that was lost or stolen.[1] Deep question for you: Do you ever feel like the essence of who you were originally created to be was taken from you by a circumstance or situation that was out of your control? I believe every person can answer yes to this, and that is why by definition recovery applies to us all. We all need to recover from the hurt of something— abuse, abandonment, codependency, someone's projection of their pain on us, or something else. We all need to recover from a habit or addiction that we or a loved one has dealt with that has impacted us in some way. We all need to recover from a hang-up that affects our attitudes in a negative way and impacts how we cope with people or hard situations such as anger, fear, depression, or unforgiveness.

All of us have experienced hardship, pain, and trauma. I wish people were exempt from this, but the truth is, we all have experienced some sort of trauma in our lifetimes. We all have had something disturbing happen to us emotionally, mentally, or physically that we need to recover from—maybe at the hands or words of a family member, spouse, clergy leader, or friend. Or perhaps from a more collective experience like a natural disaster or COVID-19, which injures our capacity to function normally. If our emotional response is impacting us in a negative way, over time this can cause a chronic problem. When this escalates, people may experience sleep disturbance, anxiety, or depression. Part of recovery work is learning to gain control over the traumatic event and figure out ways to manage and deal with those memories. When we are triggered, we need tools to deal with the negative emotional response we are having, which can lead to greater self-control, peace of mind, and stronger connections with others, and can even lessen the flashbacks.

Perhaps your innocence was lost or stolen from you as a child—if you were exposed to pornography or touched inappropriately. Maybe you were taken advantage of by a person in your life who had power over you and forced you to do unimaginable things. Through the recovery process, we can take back the power over our choices and autonomy over our bodies that were taken the moment trauma occurred. In recovery we learn that abuse is not our fault, that we could not control another person's choice to abuse, and it becomes easier to stop living in the shame that we were in that position in the first place.

Maybe you have experienced the loss of a loved one or divorced the person you thought you were going to spend the rest of your life with. Perhaps now you feel abandoned, angry at God, and utterly disappointed with the way your life has turned out. I'm so sorry for your loss, for the grief and pain. Life is unbearable and unfair at times, and recovery tools help us deal with the disappointment and grief we face across our lifetimes.

Maybe you are fearful of the future because you have experienced job loss and can't seem to get on your feet financially. You're not alone in this. Not only have rising costs of living across towns and cities of every size not been matched by pay raises in jobs across every sector of society, but the global COVID-19 crisis has resulted in an economic downturn. I wonder if today you might feel fear over the future, about how you and your family will survive.

As you can see, we cannot live our lives without injury. We need help to manage our healing and recovery. There are many ways we can categorize trauma in terms of how it affects us individually. Trauma is subjective and has its own spectrum, from exposure to chronic and/or complex disorders. A licensed psychologist is the best resource to determine where you fall on that spectrum and assist you with the path forward.

A Word to Women

Women carry an emotional and social load to be perfect, raise kids, work, and keep the house together. We lose ourselves in all we are trying to be. There is often an unfair expectation and burden, as well as a heavier mental and emotional load, on women to successfully manage a work and home life that is unmanageable. Christian women feel this pressure from the church as well. Sixty percent of the church is women, with the majority of volunteer roles staffed by females.[2] From this perspective, it's easy to see why women tend to try hard, try harder, burn out and crash, then start all over again. With no solutions in sight and no tools to ease guilt, deal with the past, or create healthy rhythms at home and work, we feel helpless to change. Not addressing what made us crash in the first place leads to coping mechanisms that are at minimum unhelpful, at maximum harmful.

We muscle through pain and transition in our lives, ignoring their impact on us as we pick up the broken pieces of our lives and faith. With our hands full, we start the cycle all over again. The problem is, many times our hands are full of anxieties, toxic rhythms and ways of relating, and burdens that need to be released. Then we try to start a new season and struggle because our arms are full, and we have the capacity to carry only so

> It's easy to see why women tend to try hard, try harder, burn out and crash, then start all over again.

much. Erykah Badu wrote a wonderful song called "Bag Lady" that expresses this idea.[3] When women run out of hands, they start picking up bags and backpacks, stuffing all their things in there without realizing the loads they carry are killing them.

For the sake of this illustration, picture putting a brick in your bag for every painful or traumatic life experience you encounter along the way. This can be a perceived or real personal failure, job loss, abuse, death of a loved one, or something else. By the time you are a young adult, you may already have a bag on your back, full of weight you can barely carry. Think about yourself as an adult and add a brick to your bag for your career pursuits, another for the stress of providing for yourself or your family, and another if you are married and are now carrying the weight of a growing relationship. Before you know it, you are carrying so much you can't walk through life without developing unhealthy ways of living. But if you learn to unload along the way as life brings new stresses and weight, you have the capacity to carry your bag without breaking down under the pressure.

I wish I would have known this in my early years. When I married at age twenty-two, my backpack was already so full that I could barely carry it. It felt like that thing weighed more than I did. Men experience this too. Just like women, without tools, without unloading baggage, they, too, can succumb to the danger of breaking down and using unhealthy coping mechanisms to deal with their stress. Adulting is hard, relationships are hard, growth is hard, recovering from failure is hard! I get it. Especially if we don't have healthy examples of how to do it.

Renewal is possible as we step out of denial and shame, into reality and recovery. Now let's talk about the thing that hinders us from taking that step: fear.

CHAPTER 6

Reframe Your Fear

As I mentioned earlier, day 38 of rehab will forever continue to speak to me as my day of reckoning. It marked a radical change in my thinking and in the trajectory of my life. It all started when I was presented with another gift of confrontation that was needed but I didn't necessarily want to have. Hindsight is 20/20 because it didn't feel like a gift at the time. I met with my psychiatrist that day, and he asked me the question again: "Do you believe you have a problem with alcohol?" My response was the same stubborn answer of no, though deep down inside I was beginning to realize that fear of facing the reality of my situation was driving my denial, while truth was loosening the grip of denial in my mind.

My psychiatrist's response shocked me as he proceeded to pull up my file on his computer and began reading out loud to me all the things my husband had shared and that I had admitted to in my intake regarding my behaviors and how I abused alcohol. He listed them: drinking to the point of blackout, hiding alcohol in water bottles, drinking and driving, not remembering events of the day while I was under the influence. Worst of all, he reminded me of the issues I was having in my marriage and the pain I was causing my loved ones. What he said next felt like a punch in the gut. He said, "Irene, if it walks like a duck, talks like a duck, then it is a duck!" This was *one* truth of my reality. My pushback was to point out the *other* reality of my situation, which was that I was doing everything the doctors recommended and I was a good student of all I was learning, I was a good mom, and I was a good person! I tried to convince him that I couldn't be an alcoholic if I was a good person. What I really feared was facing the fact that both of my realities were true. I was a good person with a purpose in life who loved her husband and children, but I also had a problem with alcohol that was about to wreck my life if I didn't acknowledge it.

His directness and harsh way of communicating with me was the much-needed shock to my system to finally change my stinking shame-based denial. I burst into tears and ran out of the session and spent the rest of the day talking to any available counselor who would listen to me cry and complain about how mean and accusatory he had been. They graciously empathized with me about the hurt I felt but did not share agreement with my thought that I was not an alcoholic. The counselors just let me be with my emotions of hurt, anger, and shame until they finally passed and I was calm enough to get back to my daily routine. The deathly grip of denial was loosening.

Will + Way = Win

"Where there is a will there is a way" is a common adage. Once our will comes into alignment with the decision to get well and do the work to get free, there is always a way out, and the end result of all the work we do to get free will establish a sure win in our lives. We win when we choose to try a different way. There are many ways we can get well. It's critical we examine ourselves and be true to our needs and research adequately the way that suits us. There is nothing new under the sun! Someone else has been there and done that and can show us the way out of our valley.

Shame can make us feel like we are deeply flawed, alone, exposed. Fear held me back from facing the shame of my recovery, but I was encouraged by those around me to consider myself brave for facing my fear of labeling myself an alcoholic. See myself as brave? Yes, it was sinking in as my mind began the work of wrapping itself around the concept of how much courage it took for me to admit my alcoholism. The payoff for getting clean doesn't feel like a payoff at all initially. When I entered rehab, I felt I had only two options: die in my addiction or just die. But the reframing work in my mind unlocked the truth of my reality. My two options were to die in my addiction or make a choice to live. I chose to live authentically and honestly the moment I stopped negotiating fear and pain and perpetuating codependency and manipulating myself and others with lame reasoning and excuses. The question was whether I had the will, desire, or "want to" to recover. I didn't initially, but it came eventually. I want to live. If not drinking means I live, then I give up. I surrender my fight to keep alcohol in my life. When we surrender our will, we find the "want to" we have been missing. With the help of God's grace and mercy, I am now able to believe the truth that it's not up to me to fix my messy life. It's up to me to surrender my mess to Jesus so He can strengthen me with His grace.

Let's consider 2 Corinthians 12:9 again, but in the Amplified

---

The question was whether I had the will, desire, or "want to" to recover. I didn't initially, but it came eventually.

Version, to expand our understanding of the exchange involved in surrendering our will to God's: "My grace is sufficient for you [My lovingkindness and My mercy are more than enough—always available—regardless of the situation]; for [My] power is being perfected [and is completed and shows itself most effectively] in [your] weakness."

Will + Way = Win. If we have the will to surrender, God is the way that will give us grace and strength, and the win is that we walk in abundance of joy, peace, and happiness regardless of our situations and what life will continue to throw at us. This is the formula I have found to walk in freedom. In John 1:16 God's Word promises us, "For from his fullness we have all received, grace upon grace" (ESV). My prayer for you is that He would heap grace upon grace on you as you continue to read the pages of this book. Grace upon grace for your journey to freedom.

Fear = Tension = Pain

We transition in life with no tools. We get pregnant and get super excited about the baby that is coming but forget that pregnancy is ten months long in reality. For many it is full of fear of the future, morning sickness, swollen body parts, random pain, and discomfort for what seems like forever. Then when labor hits and the child is about to come forth, we experience labor pains. Contractions indicate this baby is coming out! I can attest, having been there on three occasions, that the transition phase of labor is the worst part. The intensity of the pain feels unbearable, and women begin to question whether they have the strength to continue pushing the baby out.

What if you normalized the pain of transition? What if you didn't freak out when the pain of each contraction to push forth your purpose hit? What if your perspective shifted to focusing on the promise and using tools to breathe through the pain and let go of fear?

I remember learning in Lamaze class that Fear = Tension = Pain. We were taught to address the fear by becoming aware of what is happening in our bodies. When we become aware of what is happening in our bodies, we can relax because we know what we are experiencing is normal and necessary for the baby to be born. In Lamaze we learned systematic ways to breathe through the pain to relieve tension. The pain would become bearable, and we could get through it and push out the baby. We can use this same concept to approach things we fear.

One method involves asking questions that provoke us to critical thinking to find solutions to our problems. My counselor uses this technique with me to help train my brain not to panic when I get stuck in fear while reacting to trauma. In one of my counseling sessions post-rehab, I began to describe to her the feelings of anxiety and fear I experienced when I thought about moving my family to a new home. She asked me to explore the things I was afraid of and list them. After doing so, we went down the list, and I negotiated with myself over whether it was a valid fear and decided what I was going to do with it. If the fear was valid, what would be my solution to the fact that, indeed, what I was fearing could play out in my life?

I feared the stress of moving, especially the stress it would put on the kids. Would they be okay with change? Would they make new friends? Would we be accepted in the new community? Would moving make them as insecure as it made me in my own childhood experience? Would they deal with anxiety the way I do as a result? Facing each fear one at a time, I began to come up with solutions for each. My children's reality did not have to be like my own PTSD from moving often without the emotional support or tools to deal with change. I had new tools I could apply to help them feel secure and process change in a healthy way. I began to process out loud, and write down as well, that I would prepare my kids for the move by driving them through the community and visiting their new school and teachers before their first day so they could get the lay of the land, teachers, and students. We would talk through how they felt about the move and what they were most excited about. If they had any fears, we would address those fears together, as a family, so they felt supported and validated in their feelings.

My trauma-based relationship with change began to be healed, and my mind was transformed and renewed by this practical exercise for facing my fears. Catastrophizing an outcome is not helpful to any of us; it's an unnecessary stress that causes underlying anxiety. Are you ready to stop catastrophizing situations and outcomes before they even happen? I have found that it is possible to stop the vicious cycle if you choose to change your stinking thinking!

Reframe Your Fear

Fear is a natural emotion that sends us the signal that danger is present. Do you ever feel like fear has you in bondage because you are stuck in fight, flight, or freeze mode? As a survivor of PTSD, I know what that is like. I feel stuck in that response day in and day out. People with PTSD have abnormal levels of stress hormones released in our bodies. Normally, when in danger, the body produces stress hormones like adrenaline to trigger a reaction in the body. This reaction, often known as the fight-or-flight reaction, helps to deaden the senses and dull pain. People with PTSD have been found to continue to produce high amounts of fight-or-flight hormones even when there's no danger. It's thought this may be responsible for the numbed emotions and hyperarousal experienced by some people with PTSD.[1]

We were not intended to stay in this response, so our nervous systems go into overload and are overworked and overstimulated. Hence the need to satiate by reaching for something to calm ourselves, like alcohol or other substances. Trauma is defined as a deeply distressing or disturbing experience, or in medicine as an injury.[2] Trauma further overwhelms the brain's ability to cope.

Understanding PTSD

I am not an expert on PTSD, but I have done significant study on it as a result of my diagnosis in 2015. I have found that the more I learn about it and its impact on me and those around me, the more I am able to be gentle with myself and not beat myself up about things that are out of my control to change. PTSD changes the brain parts involved in emotional processing.

In brain scans of people with PTSD, parts of the brain involved in emotional processing appear different from normal brains. One part of the brain responsible for memory and emotions is known as the hippocampus. In people with PTSD, the hippocampus appears smaller in size. It's thought that changes in this part of the brain may be related to fear and anxiety, memory problems, and flashbacks. The malfunctioning hippocampus may prevent flashbacks and nightmares from being properly processed, so the anxiety they generate does not reduce over time. Treatment of PTSD results in proper processing of the memories so that over time the flashbacks and nightmares gradually disappear.[3] While PTSD is not curable, with proper treatment we can improve our quality of life by changing our responses to stimuli when triggered.

Bessel van der Kolk, MD, author of *The Body Keeps the Score—Brain, Mind, and Body in the Healing of Trauma*, wrote the following in a chapter titled "Healing from Trauma: Owning Yourself":

> Nobody can "treat" a war, or abuse, rape, molestation, or any other horrendous event, for that matter; what has happened cannot be undone. But what *can* be dealt with are the imprints of the trauma on the body, mind, and soul: the crushing sensation in your chest that you may label as anxiety or depression; the fear of losing control; always being alert for danger or rejection; the self-loathing; the nightmares and flashbacks; the fog that keeps you from staying on task and from engaging fully in what you are doing; being unable to fully open your heart to another human being.[4]

He went on to say,

> Trauma robs you of the feeling that you are in charge of yourself. . . . The challenge of recovery is to reestablish ownership of your body and your mind—of yourself. This means feeling free to know what you know and to feel what you feel without becoming overwhelmed, enraged, ashamed, or collapsed.

For most people this involves (1) finding a way to become calm and focused, (2) learning to maintain that calm in response to images, thoughts, sounds, or physical sensations that remind you of the past, (3) finding a way to be fully alive in the present and engaged in the people around you, (4) not having to keep secrets from yourself, including secrets about ways you have managed to survive.[5]

STOP

As you do research and hopefully consider working with a professional, I want to leave you with a quick tool. Instead of leaning on my addiction when I feel fear or am in fight, flight, or freeze mode, I have learned to STOP.

S—Stop . . . pause.

T—Take a deep breath.

O—Observe how I am feeling in the moment and inventory what is going on inside me. *What am I feeling and experiencing? What emotions and memories are coming up?*

P—Proceed with the plan of how I will deal with what I am experiencing. Pray, talk with someone, reality-check the thought, or affirm myself with the truth with a simple statement like "I am safe" or "I am enough."[6]

Acknowledging fear in the moment while not allowing it to overwhelm you is a skill that can be developed over time. Take a moment to reflect on what fears you may have that are impacting your quality of life. How are they affecting the way you live day to day?

From 2001 to 2012, there was a TV show called *Fear Factor* in which contestants would face their ultimate fears. I am not sure why on earth they would want to put themselves in this position except that maybe they thought exposure to their fear would cure them of it. Being put in a glass chamber full of rats is not what I would consider an effective way of overcoming a fear of rats; rather it would only create more trauma and PTSD! What is your fear factor? Where in your life can you consider reframing your fear? Now ask yourself what would happen if you saw things differently. What would happen if that fear came true? Answer the question. By exposing yourself to your worst fear created in your mind, you can walk yourself through a process of desensitization to the fear over time. (Shameless counseling plug: it may be a good idea to start this type of work with a counselor before you attempt to do it on your own. Walking through your fears with a professional counselor is freeing!)

Take a moment next time you are triggered and remember God's love for you. If 1 John 4:18 says that God's love "expels all fear" (NLT), then we can meditate and get a picture in our minds of His love showering over us and keeping us safe to combat the trigger moment. God loves us with an everlasting love. When He fills us with love, fear has to leave! Getting that picture in my mind helps me fully experience God and kick fear in the face. Now it's your turn.

CHAPTER 7

Reframe Your Identity

William Shakespeare's character Polonius in *Hamlet* made famous the words "To thine own self be true." How can you be true to yourself if you don't know yourself? To be your authentic self is to be who you are no matter where you are or who you are around, to be the same in every environment. That includes social media! Trying to be anyone other than yourself is exhausting! But to be your authentic self and to be true to yourself, you must first know yourself.

Self-Awareness

Understanding who we are, why we think and act the way we do, and how we give and receive love is something that has always fascinated me. When we begin to have a better understanding of human behavior—how we are wired—we can navigate our relationships with more grace, empathy, and objectivity. I am passionate about seeing others thrive when understanding who they are, and then applying that in their relationships.

A plethora of assessments are available to help people grow in their understanding of their true selves. Self-awareness is a critical component of becoming a functional adult with a healthy relationship with oneself and others. Who doesn't want to be the best version of themselves? Some of my favorite assessments are the Enneagram, 5 Love Languages, StrengthsFinder, Working Genius, DISC Assessment, and Myers-Briggs Type Indicator. By using these tools, we can learn a lot about how we are naturally designed, wired, and gifted. They help us understand how we communicate, filter our experiences, and best learn. Awareness of our natural giftings has value because we then can engage in activities and careers that fuel us (because they align with our interests and abilities) rather than drain us (because we aren't wired to do them). For example, if you are an extrovert and don't work with a team or around people, you will eventually be bored in your job, and this is a misery you can avoid if you are aware of the environments where you would thrive and be happy. True introverts recharge alone, while extroverts recharge around people. Are you an introvert or an extrovert? I define myself as both, and there is a term for it—*ambivert*.

You may be an ambivert if you have both introvert and extrovert traits. You love social gatherings, but you crave time alone; you can work independently or in a group and be super productive. You have a love-hate relationship with social media, can blend well with a range of personalities, and are comfortable in most environments. That is so me! I understand myself and now know that it is not a bad thing to be wired the way I am wired. I cannot be my best and truest self if I don't know how to recharge and refuel and honor what I need to be healthy and happy in my day-to-day choices and activities. Learning to be self-aware is critical in recovery because understanding our emotions and thinking leads us to better understand our behaviors. This can prove mission critical in recovery because realizing how our behaviors impact others forces us to be honest and accountable, which helps us stay sober.

Why Ignorance Is Not Bliss

If we want to grow, we must also acknowledge what we *don't* know. Anthony de Mello, an Indian Jesuit priest and psychotherapist, said, "Wisdom tends to grow in proportion to one's awareness of one's ignorance."[1]

How do you know what you don't know? You may also be wondering, *How does one change things they don't see are dysfunctional?* Perhaps you have a blind spot. Or maybe you're starting to realize that you've functioned so much on autopilot that you've been unaware of your own emotional disarray. You can start with what seems simple and small: prayer. Ask God to search your heart and reveal anything that needs to be addressed. Pray the prayer of the psalmist in Psalm 139:23–24: "Search me, O God, and know my heart; test me and know my anxious thoughts. Point out anything in me that offends you, and lead me along the path of everlasting life" (NLT).

> If we want to grow, we must also acknowledge what we *don't* know.

In their book *The Road Back to You*, Ian Morgan Cron and Suzanne Stabile describe their journey of self-discovery, often referring to how ignorance of themselves hurt not only them but also others. When we stay in ignorance of how we see the world, our past wounds, our belief systems, and how they have shaped us, we become prisoners of our history. When we aren't aware of our distorted view of the world, through how our wounds shaped us, Cron and Stabile say we are walking through life on autopilot. Our survival mechanisms can keep us asleep, and we become accustomed to making the same mistakes over and over, completely unaware of how our past impacts present behaviors. Our ignorance of ourselves can hurt us and hinder our relationships with God and others. The authors encourage us to become knowledgeable of ourselves so we can relate with the world and God in the way we were created to, rather than the learned ways that we may not realize are dysfunctional. They use the Enneagram assessment as a tool of self-discovery to get back to being the person God created us to be.[2]

I have found the Enneagram to be an amazing tool that benefits us personally, relationally, and professionally. (I know, I know, you've seen all the memes on social media about all these types of assessments, but stick with me.) The Enneagram can help us understand our wiring both positively and negatively. It also helps us develop more of a compassion for those we are in relationship with as we better understand their internal wiring and see things from their point of view. There is a reason they behave the way they do and a reason you behave, think, and act the way you do. This has more to do with the way people are wired, their experience and upbringing, than anything personal we make up about the behaviors of those around us. I am a 9 on the Enneagram, which is the peacemaker. The story I told myself was that there was something wrong with me because I naturally desire to give people the benefit of the doubt, even to a fault sometimes. At times people would walk all over me and take advantage of how agreeable I was.

I chose not to assert myself because the message the wounded Irene heard was that asserting yourself was wrong or bad. Peacemakers under stress become anxious and worried, testy and defensive, their minds racing, as internal anxiety increases. My aha moment came when I realized I would have more control over my anxiety if I would reframe the way I handle stress. Practically, through understanding my natural bent to worry, I began to meditate on scriptures to calm me down. I took control of my thought life to decrease the anxiety I felt in my belly. Philippians 4:6–7 says, "Do not be anxious about anything, but in every situation, by prayer and petition, with thanksgiving, present your requests to God. And the peace of God, which transcends all understanding, will guard your hearts and your minds in Christ Jesus."

Some of the qualities about myself that I once looked at unfavorably as weaknesses can be strengths if I lean into a more holistic perspective. For example, peacemakers have a tendency for people pleasing, but they are also good mediators, helping everyone to get along. Men and women with this personality type are peaceful and pleasant to be around, accepting and diplomatic, empathetic and caring, steady, accepting, and agreeable. I used to view this aspect of myself as codependency. Yes, there are times when I unknowingly veer toward the negatives of my personality, and I can easily slip into codependent behaviors and thinking. But now that I am aware of what dysfunctional codependent behaviors are, I can hold myself accountable to see myself and others with greater clarity. Peacemaking is a strength. Matthew 5:9 says, "Blessed [spiritually calm with life-joy in God's favor] are the makers *and* maintainers of peace, for they will [express His character and] be called the sons of God" (AMP).

My husband and I are polar opposites. He is a gregarious 7 on the Enneagram who functions with plenty of attributes of the 8. A 7 wants to have fun, is creative and full of personality, while 8s take charge. They are typically straightforward and assertive. I used to see only the negatives of his wiring. I put him in a box of being controlling and "too much" because he was always dreaming about what could be, with a desire to take risks. This brought me much anxiety for most of our marriage. I resented him for being himself. How crazy is that? I'm sure you can relate to wanting others to be more like you so you can trust them and feel safe and secure.

When Jimmy and I intentionally took time to learn how we were wired and shared these attributes with each other, we were able to understand more honestly how our behaviors impacted one another. We took ownership over our own growth process. As we did, we began to accept each other and the aspects of our personalities that we once framed as bad. We now use them for the good of strengthening our union. I can count on Jimmy to be assertive in decision-making and protecting our family, and he makes life so much more fun with his humor. He balances my indecisive nature with his strong ability to make decisions. He has accepted that I am a natural mediator, a role that benefits our union because I see things in a way that brings harmony to situations that would typically trigger him to react versus respond. I bring another point of view that he listens to now and considers as he processes how he will proceed and respond to a situation. We leverage each other's strengths and cover each other's weaknesses in a way that ultimately makes us a great team and strengthens our union of marriage. In marriage two completely different people can indeed become one if we are equally committed to the process of self-discovery. "This explains why a man leaves his father and mother and is joined to his wife, and the two are united into one" (Genesis 2:24 NLT).

Seeking understanding about who you are isn't just for married people. Knowing how you're wired, what you're good at (and not good at), helps you accept yourself. Acceptance releases shame and makes us less prone to hiding, pretending, and withholding in our relationships. It's also easier to accept others as they are and engage with them in healthier, more meaningful ways.

In our Western world, our identity can be wrapped up in what we look like, what we have, what we do, and who we know. Rather than basing our identity in possessions, performance, or people, we can reframe our view of our identity by embracing that we are made in the image of God, crafted by Him, and owned by Him. Jesus Christ lives in us! Paul wrote in Colossians 1:27, "God has chosen to make known among the Gentiles the glorious riches of this mystery, which is Christ in you, the hope of glory." True identity is found in whose you are and who God says you are. When we accept Jesus as Savior, we take on His identity and we belong to Him. We can choose to see ourselves not as ordinary or less than but as children of the living God. When we walk in the assurance of our identity being in Jesus Christ, we reframe our misconstrued view of our identity. We can exchange false reality and confusion for freedom and peace.

Identity

Who am I? What was I created for? We ask these fundamental questions, longing for answers to which we can cling. They inherently show up in early childhood when we look to people around us, such as parents, teachers, coaches, and peers, to determine our worth, value, and place in life. We desire to fit in and belong. We look externally for answers to our questions about our identity rather than internally.

As early as I can remember, I struggled with my identity. This is true for many, if not all of us. *Who am I and what was I created to do? Do I fit in? Where do I belong?* These are questions we ask ourselves. We question our sense of place in this big world. Many psychologists believe that identity formation is one of the most important conflicts human beings face.

Our go-to tends to be finding identity in others, such as our parents and siblings, extended family, spouses, or friends we hang around with. We look to others in early childhood, especially our parents, to affirm that we are good, but what if our parents don't affirm us for some reason? As adults we may look to what we *do* in our career, parenting, serving in the church, and so forth for our identity. The problem with that is these are all external things, yet identity is discovered from within. Who are you beneath the fear and the shame? Who are you past what you do? Who are you when things like jobs or people transition out of your life or get taken away by job layoffs or death? What happens when you become an empty nester, underprepared for the emptiness in your home and heart, left with just yourself? If we struggle to know and identify who we are in ourselves, life events can create identity crises in us.

A poor sense of self-worth (also known as poor self-esteem) occurs when you come to believe that you have little value or worth. This often occurs when key people in your life are critical of you or when you are perfectionistic and critical of yourself.[3] I tend to be my own worst critic, picking apart my features, my hair, my intelligence, my skill as a public speaker, my parenting—the list goes on and on.

When I was in second grade, my dad walked me to my classroom as I was arriving late due to a doctor's appointment. When I opened the door to the classroom, all the students whipped their heads around and stared at my dad and me with perplexed expressions on their faces. I grew insecure as I put my coat in my cubby and walked toward my seat, heat rising in my face, embarrassed from all the looks I was receiving. After class a boy asked me why my dad was white and my mom was Black. I told him I had no idea. Was there something wrong with that? Based on what he and the others said about me, it was bad. *Boom!* The start of low self-esteem over my race, skin color, and hair texture began.

Growing up biracial, half Black (Zambian) and half Caucasian (American), made me African American, right? I was confused and struggled to understand what category I belonged in, what race I belonged to. I was born abroad, but my dad was a US citizen, so did that make me American, and did that mean I was to identify as Black American? Was biracial a category at all? What race was I going to identify with? I struggled to identify because everyone seemed so different from me. This lack of understanding my identity perpetuated my shame while deepening my insecurities.

Many of us have experienced a bully in our lives. Someone who used name-calling or slander to one-up themselves, putting us down to feel better about themselves. I am sure someone has hurled hurtful or verbally abusive words at you. Anything less than nurturing can go into the category of abuse. When we allow untruths, divisive rumors, or attacks on our character and reputation to define our identity, we are in danger of sliding down the self-esteem scale. We must know for ourselves who we are at the core so that, when circumstances or people tell us otherwise, we can combat that with truth and not be shaken emotionally or believe a lie about ourselves.

A strategy I have given my children is to picture themselves every morning before they leave the house for school with a permeable bubble around them. Words can flow in and out of this bubble, and it serves as a boundary for protection. Boundaries are necessary, and I didn't grow up learning how to set them, so I was sure to teach this skill to my kids as I learned it. I let them know that they get to decide what comes into their bubble. Every time someone, whether an adult, like a teacher or coach, or a peer, says something to them, they catch the words on the outside of the bubble, examine the words against what they believe about themselves, then decide if they will take them into the bubble. If the words have truth, they may enter; if they are untrue or hurtful or an attack, my children shut them out and let them rebound to the person who said them. When they practice this boundary technique, they are affirming for themselves that the other person's words have nothing to do with them. Rather, those words are a projection of the way that person feels about themselves. The words hold no truth, so my children will not allow them to be their truth.

When I discovered that my identity was rooted in God, something changed in me. Having my identity in God reframed the way I viewed myself as I turned to the truth of God's Word to find out how God sees me. Being a child of God meant in simple terms that I was His daughter. God's daughter. A child of God (Romans 8:14; 2 Corinthians 6:18; Galatians 3:26). But what if we have a skewed filter of what it means to be a child of God because our experience with our earthly parents has been nothing short of disappointment, abandonment, neglect, abuse, and mistreatment? Maybe your parents didn't know how to be emotionally supportive or struggled with mental health issues or addiction themselves and didn't have the knowledge, ability, or mental capacity to be what you needed them to be. This makes viewing God as Father challenging for some. How do we receive God's love if we don't trust Him or see Him as safe?

We can turn to countless scriptures to meditate on and think of often when we fall into a self-esteem rut or shame attack, struggling with how we feel about ourselves. They will not only redirect our thinking but reprogram it as well. Ephesians 2:10 assures us, "We are God's masterpiece. He has created us anew in Christ Jesus, so we can do the good things he planned for us long ago" (NLT). The psalmist wrote that we are "fearfully and wonderfully made" (Psalm 139:14). And we can take comfort in knowing that God chose us; we did not choose Him (John 15:16). My prayer for you is that you dig deeper in learning more about who you are and take confidence in knowing that you were specifically designed the way you are, flaws and all, for a purpose. May you find freedom as you discover and accept your identity.

CHAPTER 8

Reframe Dysfunction

Going from dysfunction to function was and still is a challenge for our entire family. We are learning every day to call out dysfunction when we see it in one another and problem-solve together to process through it. My children call me out for codependent behaviors, such as when my response to where we are going to eat or go on vacation is about what everyone else wants. They ask me, "Mom, are you sure you have considered what you want and that you aren't just doing this for us?" They remind me that what I want matters too, and that they are open to compromise so we all get something we want rather than sulk and be miserable because we didn't really want to do what we agreed on.

The Impact of Codependency

We all have a little codependency in us because of dysfunctional childhood experiences. This is reflected in our relationship with self and our relationship with others. Pia Mellody wrote in *Facing Codependence*, "Codependent people have difficulty experiencing appropriate levels of self-esteem, setting functional boundaries, owning and expressing their own reality, taking care of the adult needs and wants, and experiencing and expressing their reality moderately."[1]

When we dig around our past, we find the root issues of our negative behaviors. We find why we do what we do, why we act the way we do, why we treat others the way we do, and why we allow other people to treat us the way they do. Taking time to dig up the answers and work through creating our new normal is messy, exhausting, scary, and difficult, and it can feel like we are all alone doing it sometimes. This is exactly why most people don't do the work to get healthy and free. We stay the same, miserable, and in prisons of our own making.

Codependency was my own personal prison for far too long. My life had been about pleasing people, and I had a lack of boundaries both internally and externally. I felt I needed to be there for people and make them happy, and therefore I wouldn't share my needs because I felt like I was supposed to be strong and perfect. I couldn't experience appropriate levels of self-esteem and lived primarily with low self-esteem, feeling severely inadequate and believing I would never be enough. Because I had so much difficulty owning my own reality and expressing it, I took on or became agreeable to the reality of those around me. Nearly every time I was around others, I became chameleon-like, taking on the nature of whomever or whatever I was around. Acknowledging my own needs and wants was a struggle, and I lacked the ability to take care of myself because I didn't think I was worthy of care, rest, and investment. I had a total lack of self-worth, and I secretly resented everyone around me and felt they were somehow to blame for my misery. I was always the victim, playing the blame game. Shame seemed magnified in me, and I felt crazy and irrational in my thinking. I was either unreactive or overreactive to situations in my life. Why did I feel so crazy? Because I was codependent!

People who deal with codependency typically do not understand the magnitude of it and how it impacts our happiness, mental health, quality of relationships, and self-esteem. Psychologists debate whether codependency can be called a disease. If the dictionary defines a disease as a particular quality, habit, or disposition regarded as adversely affecting a person or group of people, then codependency can be categorized as a disease. My life was out of control emotionally, which ultimately led to being out of control physically as well when I medicated my pain with alcohol and became dependent. Could it be that codependency is the root of my addiction? In my experience, when I removed alcohol, I was left to deal with the symptoms and many consequences of codependency in my recovery journey. So yes, I believe codependency is the root of my drinking. I also believe many people are dealing with codependency in their lives and relationships but don't know how to identify it, let alone address it.

How does this destructive situation arise? Psychotherapist Dariane Pictet said:

> Codependents have learned to value themselves as a helper. When you grow up with alcoholic parents, around someone narcissistic or with a mother that puts herself first, you will learn at 2 or 3 years old that you have to serve the mother or father and that's how you get the brownie points, that's how you get recognition and have some kind of safety in the relationship.[2]

I meet people all the time whose lives are out of control and spiraling downward because of codependency, and they can't seem to put a finger on what it is that is going on and causing them such emotional turmoil. They are being manipulated by someone else financially or emotionally, or are inappropriately dependent on someone else, and/or esteem themselves by being the helper. These people are accepting excuses for someone else's bad behaviors and bailing them out of their problems, not allowing them to experience consequences for their choices.

All these scenarios impact a codependent person's mental health negatively. Those who are manipulating or taking advantage of you are violating boundaries. They may not even be aware of what they are doing because often the motivation is in their subconscious. They are not bad, but if you allow the relationship to continue, you will feed into the dysfunctional codependent relationship. Becoming aware of your own needs, thoughts, and feelings, and being able to separate those from another's needs, thoughts, and feelings helps draw boundary lines where enmeshment has occurred. Then you can begin speaking up about your needs and wants, as well as how you want and deserve to be treated, to improve your situation and relationships. Learn to say no. You know your limits, and it's okay to communicate them.

In my experience, therapists have a hard time treating the symptoms of codependency with the little information available, and few people understand it and deal with it effectively. They treat all the symptoms but not the root issue. For years it felt like I was shooting a BB gun in a war where the enemy had military weapons. We don't stand a chance! Life stressors, abuse, and dysfunction are multiplying in our society, yet the tools and awareness needed to deal with codependency are moving at a snail's pace.

If you are struggling with codependency, you probably feel like you do more for others than for yourself. This perpetuates the codependency symptoms of resentment and victim mentality. We believe it's everyone else's fault that we are miserable and not doing what we want with our lives. It is always about serving your kids or your husband's career endeavors, while ignoring your own desires to live out your unique purpose in life. This was me for years because I made it my primary goal in life to support my husband in his ministry at the church. As he gave what seemed like all his time to pastoring people, I never communicated that I needed him to invest in me and our marriage. Sometimes I just needed help with the kids or for him to help with laundry or dishes. We both worked full-time, but I did not communicate what I needed in our partnership while raising the kids together. I quickly got burned out and angry at him for not making us enough of a priority. This sent me into the resentment cycle that ate away at our love relationship. I created my own misery by not facing my codependent behaviors of being needless/wantless and focused on caring for others while I was secretly dying of resentment.

Where are you on the self-esteem continuum? Are you aware of your highs and lows in your self-esteem and what triggers those extremes? Do you like yourself? Why or why not? Do you take care of yourself appropriately and communicate what you need and want to do that? If you want to live a meaningful and happy life, then it's time to face codependency and do the work to get free. You must identify areas where you are dysfunctional in your relationship with yourself and others, set functional boundaries, and learn how to esteem yourself and care for yourself appropriately.

Doing these things is challenging when you are taking care of a medically ill loved one or an aging parent who is unable to care for themselves, or if you have to be there for others who are going through grief or hardship. Such situations can be overwhelming even if you have the best of intentions. We want to be there for people we love, and we most certainly can be. However, we must be mindful to take care of ourselves in the midst of caring for others and ask for help or a time-out if we need it. We can't care for others unless we care for ourselves first.

Recovery from codependency is an uphill battle and is something I will deal with for the rest of my life. I have accepted this. I have also reframed what I thought was a death sentence as an opportunity to exercise my new tools to live a happier, healthier life—one that I deserve and have always desired.

My hope is that your new awareness of the destructive nature of codependency and how it steals your joy fuels you to learn more about how it may be sabotaging your life and relationships.

Emotional Intelligence

Have you ever seen others have pointless road rage and fly off the handle with uncontrollable anger? Just key in "road rage" in a YouTube search, and you will have a field day and likely some good laughs over all the out-of-control people who make fools of themselves by lashing out in anger. They are caught on camera doing and saying things I am sure they regret that are forever on the internet! Many of these situations are avoidable if only we learn to recognize and deal with our emotions moderately in the moment we are triggered. Sometimes a lack of emotional intelligence looks like a boss at work who not only is a bully but gives special treatment only to people they like. Perhaps you have experienced people who lack empathy showing no reaction to other people who are experiencing tremendous sadness, tragedy, or even joy. They don't respond in a way that is fitting for the emotion the other person is experiencing, and they come off cold and detached. These are examples of low emotional intelligence.

With addiction, low emotional intelligence impacts one's motivation to use a substance due to a lack of self-awareness and self-regulation. As one resource explained, "Emotional intelligence or EI is the ability to understand and manage your own emotions, and those of the people around you. People with a high degree of emotional intelligence know what they're feeling, what their emotions mean, and how these emotions can affect other people."[3]

In EI development, having the capacity to be aware of others' emotions and how they impact us is equally important. Having this understanding gives us the ability to manage our relationships effectively. A high EI helps us build stronger relationships not only at home but at our jobs and at school. It can help reduce stress and improve job satisfaction and overall happiness in life. Emotional intelligence has been proven to be a better indicator of success in performance and development of potential than having a high IQ—that is, your EI will determine your success and happiness in life more than your IQ will.

There are various models and approaches to teaching EI, but it is commonly defined by four attributes:

1. **SELF-MANAGEMENT:** You're able to control impulsive feelings and behaviors, manage your emotions in healthy ways, take initiative, follow through on commitments, and adapt to changing circumstances.

2. **SELF-AWARENESS:** You recognize your own emotions and how they affect your thoughts and behavior. You know your strengths and weaknesses and have self-confidence.

3. **SOCIAL AWARENESS:** You have empathy. You can understand the emotions, needs, and concerns of other people, pick up on emotional cues, feel comfortable socially, and recognize the power dynamics in a group or organization.

4. **RELATIONSHIP MANAGEMENT:** You know how to develop and maintain good relationships, communicate clearly, inspire and influence others, work well in a team, and manage conflict.[4]

The good news is that emotional intelligence is a skill that can be developed at any age. For me, acknowledging my emotions rather than denying them was a critical step in growing in emotional awareness and intelligence. Just as we learn dysfunction, we can unlearn it.

Experiencing the painful emotions of grief and loss is something that almost took me out at one point in my life. I expected that friends with whom I did life, having double birthday parties for our kids and sharing holidays and experiences where we laughed and cried together, would be in my life forever. That wasn't the case when our friendships got complicated. For one reason or another, they were no longer in my life. Yes, I was aware that I was experiencing pain from the loss of relationship. The problem was, I didn't know how to process that pain and move past it. This not knowing what to do was an indication of low emotional intelligence and caused an inexplicable anxiety that over time compounded into deep unhappiness and a state of hopelessness. As an emotional infant in my thirties, with no idea how to acknowledge and express what was happening inside me, stuffing and numbing was what I knew. And I thought it was working until it didn't work anymore.

Emotional Health

We need resources, practical tools, and personal stories that we can identify with and learn from to grow in emotional healing and self-awareness. Author Peter Scazzero is an incredible resource with books, podcasts, and more on the topic of emotional health and how it impacts our relationships with self and others, as well as our leadership capabilities and spirituality. In his book *Emotionally Healthy Spirituality*, Scazzero wrote, "It is not possible to be spiritually mature while remaining emotionally immature."[5] He also addressed leaders in his book *The Emotionally Healthy Leader*: "The emotionally unhealthy leader is someone who operates in a continuous state of emotional and spiritual deficit, lacking emotional maturity and a 'being *with* God' [spending time in fellowship and worship] sufficient to sustain their 'doing *for* God'" [all the activities we do in God's name, such as serving the homeless].[6]

Here are some indicators that you may be emotionally unhealthy and at risk:

- You give away the best of you, meaning you dedicate the best of your time, energy, thought, and creative efforts to others at the expense of yourself and your closest relationships.

- You are chronically overextended, meaning you do more activity for God than you invest in your relationship with God.
- You lack a sabbath rhythm and don't take enough time to value rest.
- You avoid healthy conflict, stuffing and numbing your emotions.
- You lack boundaries and live life without limits.

All these symptoms are dangerous when we are unaware of them.

Emotional Health and Rest

Something I struggle with maintaining in my emotional health journey is rest. Rest is a commandment, not a suggestion. Even God rested after He spent six days creating. What makes us think we can operate on empty and not crash and burn at some point? We can't serve others well unless we serve ourselves well. We can feel guilty and even selfish about self-care when we don't value our own worth. Self-care is not selfish—it's self-esteem! When you regard yourself well, you take care of yourself and don't feel guilty about it because you are worth it! This is something I have to tell myself daily—and I mean *daily*—to try to overcome my pattern of working so hard that I end up in burnout and emotional disarray.

If I don't keep self-care at the forefront, I am in danger of relapse. Relapse will be knocking on the door ready to pounce on me when my emotions are in turmoil and not dealt with, when I am mentally exhausted and not alert for triggers, or when my physical body is weak because I am sick. A lack of self-care makes all of us susceptible to reaching out for the unhealthy thing we are tempted to cope with.

Numerous apps are available to use as tools to improve your self-awareness. A phone app can remind us to get connected with ourselves and be mindful of what is happening in our bodies and emotions. The app I use is called Calm, and it just popped up a message as I was writing this chapter. It said, "Are you aware of what you are feeling in your body right now?" (Ha!) It reminds me to breathe deeply and release tension in mind, gut, and shoulders, where I typically store my stress. I take a moment to acknowledge my emotions and discover what they are trying to alert me to deal with.

Moderating Your Emotions

When we are stressed, it's more difficult to contain our emotions. We lash out in anger, wounding those around us and damaging our relationships, and those closest to us experience the brunt of it. Anger is a normal emotion, but if not handled properly, it can result in verbal outbursts that can be abusive and harmful to others. Awareness of the extremes in our emotions helps us regulate them. The consequences of not having control of our anger or expressing it out of moderation can cause big *T*'s or little *t*'s of trauma in those around us. Do people walk on eggshells around you? Does your family experience fear or even anxiety when you get home from work because they don't know what mood you are in? Are they afraid you'll lash out at them because you happen to be angry? Grow in your EI by making an honest evaluation of how your mood impacts those around you. Ask for feedback to help you step out of denial and into reality of how your anger affects them. Apologize quickly and make amends where necessary to begin healing those you may have hurt in your anger.

We owe it to our loved ones to take care of ourselves so they can experience the best of us. It may mean taking a few minutes in the car to finish a phone call so that when you enter the home you can give your full, undivided attention to your spouse or family. Maybe it means taking a moment to do deep-breathing exercises on the car ride home from a stressful day at work, or listening to worship music, going for a walk, or doing something else that relaxes you. We are responsible for doing the work to refresh and revive ourselves so we can engage in a healthy way with those we love. De-stressing ourselves and doing self-care ultimately benefits everyone around us.

As you become more self-aware in your recovery and grow in emotional intelligence, your quality of life and contentment in relationships will bear tangible results. Ask God to reveal to you the areas that need work in your emotional awareness, stress management, and other behaviors related to codependency that are not serving you well. Do the work to get free, and you are sure to live a more fulfilling life and have mutually satisfying relationships as a result. The work is worth it!

> We owe it to our loved ones to take care of ourselves so they can experience the best of us.

CHAPTER 9

Reframe Your Normal

I remember sitting on the plane to fly back home by myself on Christmas Eve, fresh out of rehab. I affirmed myself despite the tears and shame, fighting the fear of my husband, children, and community rejecting me upon my return to Maryland. I was so incredibly fragile. Like on the first day after having a cast removed from a broken limb, I gingerly and cautiously approached all my first interactions as a sober woman. Working my steps and new programming moment by moment, case by case, I faced my new reality with fear and trembling. I'd learned that if I could just get past the "firsts"—first time seeing my family, first holiday in years sober, first Sunday back with our church family—I'd enter my new reality. A reality of freedom, healing, and forgiveness.

With my phone in my hand, after not having it for forty days in rehab, I was confronted with my first of many shame attacks. I reached out to my siblings to update them that I was safe and on my way home. I failed in my response to the shame attack when

I sent a text asking them not to tell anyone I had been in rehab. Recovery is messy and imperfect, and we will stumble along the way, as I did on many occasions. As I sat in my seat on the plane, I felt hot around my neck, face, and upper chest and noticed an uncomfortable feeling in the pit of my stomach as I thought about reentry back home. I could tell by my new awareness of my emotions and connectedness with my body that those were clear signals that I was dealing with shame. I decided to apply a new technique to get through the shame I was feeling as a mother, wife, daughter, sister, friend, and pastor—on her way home from *rehab*.

I pulled out my phone and began to type out the following affirmations to remind myself of the truth:

12/24/15

I am enough.

I am worth it.

You make me brave, God.

I accept my humanity today.

I love myself.

I forgive myself.

God loves me.

Jesus is in my heart, and the Holy Spirit lives in me.

I am worthy.

His grace is sufficient for me.

My husband and children love me.

My family, friends, and church family love me.

I am a good person.

I am capable of being honest.

I am lovable.

I am a grateful recovering alcoholic.

I have a new way of living life.

It is well with my soul.

I hear Your voice again, Lord, and feel Your presence.

I am forgiven.

I'll never forget this opportunity for healing and life change.

I am grateful and hopeful.

I have joy in my heart.

Thank You, God, for a second chance.

I am sober.

I can live a sober life.

I will be gentle with Irene.

I am free.

I am perfectly imperfect.

I own my recovery.

I can live my life as a functional adult.

My recovery will not be perfect.

I am vigilant and alert, connected and anchored to God.

I am connected to my true self.

My emotions matter and deserve to be honored.

I am capable of giving and receiving love and intimacy.

I am affectionate and loving.

I am the apple of God's eye.

I am a miracle.

The question I asked myself was, *How is it possible to be sober and still enjoy my life?* To answer this question, I had to reframe the way I saw and experienced fun in my life. Mocktails over cocktails. Enjoying new sober friends and friends who still drink but value recovery and would help in supporting me to protect my own.

Cherishing moments with my family that I took for granted while I was abusing alcohol.

Every "first" is an opportunity to practice reframing shame-based thinking. It was way too easy to slip back into my old habit of allowing myself to spiral into shame, because I was familiar with this pattern of thinking. But choosing to disrupt that thinking with positivity and affirmations of truth helped me bravely face my family, friends, and new reality at home. Truth encouraged me to believe that I am loved and that my family wanted me home, sober, and well.

A psalm that is especially meaningful to me says, "I sought the LORD, and he answered me and delivered me from all my fears. Those who look to him are radiant, and their faces shall never be ashamed" (Psalm 34:4–5 ESV). When I look back at pictures from when I first got home from rehab, I can see a glow and radiance about me. Isaiah 61 is another powerful passage, and one of the things it promises is that in our trauma, abuse, and pain, we can receive double honor for our shame (v. 7). How encouraging to know that even after our mistakes, addictions, and dysfunction, God wants to give us honor for our shame. The love we receive from God and others opens up our hearts to a new and better way of life as we navigate our new normal.

Now, as I scroll through photos on my phone from those first days back at home, I see the *new me* and notice how different I look, which matched how good I felt on the inside. I wasn't faking a smile or pretending to be happy. I actually *was* happy. Despite how good I felt about my new reality, when I scrolled back and saw photos of the old Irene, I just wanted to press Delete. So I pressed Delete in my phone and on social media, erasing reminders of the old Irene, that shameful person I was before going to rehab.

My eyes were droopy in some of the
photos, and I could remember that I
was under the influence at the time the
photo was taken. I stared in disbelief at
the radical change I could see in myself

I wasn't faking a smile or pretending to be happy. I actually
was happy.

and how sick I had been in comparison to the woman I was finally
okay looking at in the mirror. This moment defined my transition
from being a disgrace to surrendering to God's amazing grace that
rescued me from myself and my addiction.

A New Normal

Once our mind's eye is open to the joy and possibilities of a new way
of life, the old ways of thinking, of relating to people and God, and
of coping with stress just aren't going to work anymore. I got off the
plane and ran to the baggage claim area to meet my kids after the
torture of not seeing them for forty days. We dramatically ran to
one another and embraced and cried. It felt like a scene straight out
of a Hallmark movie. I will never forget our meeting. Plus, I have
the selfie we took with the balloons they brought me to document
the moment. I don't tend to take a lot of selfies because I rather
enjoy being in the moment, but I knew that when I looked back
at that picture, it would remind me of the opportunity I had for a
second chance at a healthy relationship with my kids. That photo
helps me keep the pain near to my heart, so I don't forget how close
I was to losing them and losing my life.

Walking back into the house after the airport high, I sensed
tension rising in my body. The hole in the wall where Jimmy threw
his phone in anger in one of our arguments was a painful reminder

of the state we were in only forty days ago. The places I hid my alcohol were mocking me with shame. How was I going to cook or end my day without alcohol? As the anxiety and fear rise in us, and we start to crave our old coping mechanisms, it's important to stay present in the moment. The future can feel overwhelming. It's a struggle to believe we can live a new way. Moment by moment we overcome. Every single small decision leads to change. I survived my reentry back home, and then I kept waking up each morning and feeding my new perspective in meditation, working the steps of my program and loving myself as I practiced this new normal.

I remember attending church the first time post-rehab, wondering if anyone knew where I had been for the last month and fearing someone asking me about it. I had made up the script that my issues impacted the church negatively, even though it wasn't public what Jimmy and I had gone through. After being home for about a year or so, I began to hear of the people who had left the church. I couldn't help but feel guilt and shame, because the story I told myself was that their leaving was personal toward me in some way, and that I was responsible. I wondered if our inability to lead effectively through our crisis had created a trickle-down effect to our church. I felt I had let our congregation down, and I grieved the fact that I never showed them or allowed them to get to know the real Irene.

As I sat in church that day watching all God's people worship with abandonment and adoration, God moved in the hearts of His people, and many came to know the freeing power of Jesus Christ in that service. The revelation hit me that this was God's church, the people were ultimately His responsibility, and the weight of their lives, issues, and pain was not mine to carry. It is God's responsibility to save the lost, and mine is simply to obey Him and do my part to love and shepherd the people He sends to our church. They never belonged to me, and their transitions were their decisions for what was best for their families' needs. As I sat with that truth, it was time to apply my new tool of rehearsing affirmations instead of nursing wounds. Doing so created turnaround thoughts to snap me out of the shame that made me want to run away from my faith community.

I am not bad because of the crisis we went through. I didn't ruin the church or my family, and that guilt and shame do not belong to me. God rescued me and will use all that we have been through for good (Romans 8:28). God did not change His mind about me; He will still use me. Romans 11:29 says, "God's gifts and his call are irrevocable." God will use our family's story to save the lives of many people. As Joseph told his brothers, "You intended to harm me, but God intended it for good to accomplish what is now being done, the saving of many lives" (Genesis 50:20).

We often don't see God moving in the moment, but He is always at work in us and through us. He is always working for our good even when we don't see Him working. I was not disqualified from ministry or pastoring. In fact, my mess enhanced the call of God on my life. It was only a matter of time before God used it for good.

Intentional Decisions

Creating our new normal requires facing our "firsts" with courage. Firsts are an opportunity to begin to reframe our normal. Firsts are a big deal in life, from our first day of school, to our first date, to our first kiss. When we experience a first in life, we are nervous and fearful of the unknown. *How will things turn out? How will I respond or react when I am in my first situation while fragile and straight out of rehab? What will it be like when I see my ex for the first time since our divorce or breakup?* The tools we have, the boundaries we keep, are like guardrails that keep us from going over the edge and reverting to our old ways of responding to situations that confront us.

Reframing our new normal starts with the intent to begin behaving in a new way. Having guardrails means having accountability when approaching our firsts as we create new and healthy patterns and behaviors. We need people we can be open and honest with about our feelings, experiences, and struggles, who can guide us to safety. On those fragile first days especially, we need intentionality in all areas—friendships, counseling, weekly support groups like AA or Celebrate Recovery, a faith community and church home, honesty, and courage to be vulnerable with our needs, fears, and struggles. Getting honest with my husband about my fear of walking into my first AA meeting after rehab gave me the opportunity to receive the encouragement I needed to boost my confidence to just do it. The anxiety I felt walking into that room was so overwhelming it almost prevented me from going to get the support I needed to stay sober. Being honest about what I felt in the moment and asking for help was part of my new normal. And I liked it!

I felt stronger after I got over my first time of being honest with Jimmy about how hard it was for me to be in a restaurant and see all the alcohol around that I could not have. I was fresh in my sobriety at the time, and I noticed every cocktail, glass of wine, and liquor on display in restaurants and felt a longing to have some myself, like everyone around me. Jimmy appreciated my honesty about how I struggled with that on our first dinner out together as a sober woman and helped me from then on by asking servers to seat us at tables as far from the bar as possible. Watching the woman next to our table drink her crisp sauvignon blanc was torture. I lustfully stared at her every sip. Deep grief came over me as I watched normal drinkers around me. I felt anger and resentment in the moment that I could not drink like they were.

I shared all of this with Jimmy, and he said, "Who is this new woman who actually shares her good, bad, and ugly feelings with me? I could get used to this!" This was a glimpse into our new normal. When I was honest about still having a strong compulsion to drink, that helped Jimmy give me the support I needed. For a season, I even had to tell him that I needed to have my back to the bar when seated in a restaurant just so I didn't have to look at all the delicious bottles of wine and liquor. Yes, the cravings were almost unbearable at the beginning of my sobriety. I assumed Jimmy would still drink—after all, it was his right. I'm the one with the issue. But he said, "Why would I drink in front of you when it almost destroyed our marriage and family?" I was shocked and relieved! I felt loved, cared for, and seen by my husband. I've seen many of my friends in AA struggle with alcohol still being in their homes and wrestle with sobriety while their spouses drank. I'm so glad I didn't have to deal with that struggle.

No doubt about it—I still had a compulsion to drink, until it started to fade over time, about three years into my sobriety. Therefore, I had to approach all my first encounters with temptations with my big-kid gloves on and a heightened awareness of how easily I could slip back into old behaviors. Intentionality with being honest, transparent, and accountable were the guardrails I needed desperately to keep me on track with developing my new normal.

The first time I drove by myself was nerve-racking. Passing

by the liquor stores I used to stop at so regularly, it felt as though my car had a magnet that would draw me in, and now with my new sober mind I had to protect myself. I had to be intentional about every environment I put myself in and every decision I made post-rehab in my new normal. When staying in a hotel, I would ask for alcohol to be removed from my room before I arrived. I sometimes still do this today even though I don't have a compulsion to drink. I don't even care to be distracted by alcohol or to use energy toward it, so out of sight is out of mind, one less thing I have to think about.

These kinds of intentional daily decisions protect our sobriety and build character and habits that keep us on track in our new normal. If you struggle with porn, maybe you would consider not having certain channels available on your TV at home, and where you travel, have the hotel disable movie purchases on the TV in your room. You may also consider putting software on your phone or computer that alerts a trusted accountability partner if you attempt to visit a porn site; or block your access to such material online altogether. I have spoken to many parents who discovered their children were watching porn, and after confronting them about it, the children expressed relief when their parents put monitoring software on their devices because they were exhausted from dealing with the temptation of having porn so readily available and having to hide what they were doing.

What environments create temptation that is too difficult for you to overcome? What new boundaries or guardrails might you need to put in place to protect your sobriety? What intentional decisions can you make to stay on track in your new normal? Each first you overcome will lay the foundation for the next right decision you need to make. I felt stronger each time I experienced a first and handled a situation or relationship differently than I had in the past.

Freedom vs. Responsibility

Remember in the beginning of this book, when I talked about how our culture celebrates drinking as a normal way to relieve stress, get through parenting, or take the edge off at work or at home? This is nothing new. These scenarios have been playing out for centuries and have been deemed normal for cultures all around the world. Wine played such an important role in Greek culture that they have a god named Dionysus who is the Greek god of wine and ecstasy. In Greek mythology, he glorified debauchery and the freedom to do as one pleased in excess.[1] *You may not be as bad as the Greek god Dionysus, but you are tempted to head there.*

Like the image Dionysus signified, the culture and world around us make us believe that we have the freedom to choose and do as we please, but we also bear the responsibility to manage our choices and behavior in moderation. We have the freedom to do anything, but not everything is good for us. As 1 Corinthians 10:23 says, "'I have the right to do anything,'—but not everything is constructive." All things are lawful for me, *but* not all things are helpful or beneficial to me.

The key is to be so self-aware that we are alert to the downward slope of compulsion toward a substance or thing, so we can catch ourselves from slipping into it. Reframing *your* normal should challenge you to think about what you have deemed normal and consider whether it is beneficial for you despite what others or society is telling you is right or normal.

What the Bible Says About Addiction

As we reframe our normal, let's consider our view of what addiction means through the lens of the Bible. "The Bible has a different definition of addiction, which involves our relationship with God. Addiction is choosing or pursuing something other than God in a habitual, patterned, or repetitive way in order to meet a particular need, despite the inadequacy of the coping mechanism and the negative consequences that occur," Dr. Karl Benzio, a Christian psychologist who founded Lighthouse Network, wrote.[2]

Addiction is like idol worship in a sense, because we are giving our power over to something that is contrary to God and to what is good for us, like the Greek god Dionysus. Tension regarding addiction is spoken about in the Bible. The tension is centered around whether our devotion is rightfully oriented around God or misoriented around an idol. Second Peter 2:19 says that "people are slaves to whatever has mastered them." *Whatever enslaves you will end up mastering you*, and this is a fact. I was enslaved to my drinking, and nothing could stop me. No person. No thing. True freedom comes when we are no longer in the state of being enslaved by something. For me that involved getting help, deprogramming unhealthy patterns of thinking and responding to difficult situations and stress, going to rehab, dealing with the root issues in counseling, being around people like me who had similar goals and desires to stop abusing what was making us sick, and attending regular AA meetings to help reprogram my brain from addictive desires. In other words, breaking free didn't happen spontaneously for me. I had to work to free myself.

The drinking of wine versus holiness is yet another facet of the debate about whether alcohol is biblically acceptable. In biblical times, wine was a part of the culture as it is today, consumed at festivals and weddings like the one where Jesus' first miracle took place (turning water into wine). Wine was used for Communion and was consumed at the Last Supper. Therefore, it's easy to decide that wine is not bad for *you* and is okay to consume. This conclusion is not wrong either. After all, it's not illegal, nor is it unbiblical to drink. You have the right to drink if you choose to. But the important question to ask yourself is, "Is it beneficial for me?" You have the freedom to make that choice for yourself and the responsibility to be honest with yourself about whether drinking is okay for you. If you have difficulty moderating your drinking, or the consequences are escalating, like DUIs or blackouts, it may be time to consider a life without it. I get that this is hard. As you now know, for quite some time I could not imagine my life without alcohol. It took me a while to process that I was not missing out on a happy life by not consuming alcohol.

The Bible tells us to devote ourselves to teaching and preaching the Word of God. Acts 2:42 says the early church "devoted themselves to the apostles' teaching and to fellowship, to the breaking of bread and to prayer." If the object of our affection is rightly oriented, it can be devotion. Devotion is defined as a love, loyalty, or enthusiasm for a person, activity, or cause, as in religious worship, prayer, or observance.[3] Another meaning of devotion is religious fervor or the fact or state of being dedicated and loyal.[4] I think many clergy leaders and lay ministers get this twisted because we see serving God as a good thing. It is a good thing; however, when we are burning the candle at both ends, like many church leaders are, our serving can become destructive and unhealthy. If things are okay in moderation, maybe people are doing the opposite and burning out, filling schedules beyond capacity, and not giving appropriate time to our relationships with loved ones or God because we are too busy. Too many church leaders alienate their spouses and families because what they are doing in devotion to God becomes their priority, even over their responsibilities to the people they love most. Family members, close friends, and children can begin to feel like they are second in life, less important than the church, and may even become resentful of the church and God. Serving God is good, but not if your family or marriage is falling to the wayside.

We can glean further insight from 1 Corinthians 16:15–16: "You know that the household of Stephanas were the first converts in Achaia, and they have devoted themselves to the service of the Lord's people. I urge you, brothers and sisters, to submit to such people and to everyone who joins in the work and labors at it." Verse 15 speaks to devotion to service as God's people. The word *devoted* is used when doing ministry for God. Having a determination toward something good is great until it is out of moderation. When our lives become unbalanced as we serve God's people, this could be considered a "holy addiction." We can be addicted to good things too! We can't serve God's people if we are neglecting ourselves and our responsibilities. We can't work, work, work and neglect ourselves or our home life. Jimmy and I were guilty of this unhealthy imbalance for more than fifteen years of our marriage, and it ate away at our intimacy and connection. Instead of speaking up and asking for what I needed and wanted for our marriage, I ate resentment pie over and over, which built up over the years into undealt-with pain, fueling my use of alcohol to cope while Jimmy used food to cope. Pure insanity!

Church ministry is the field our family is in, so I reference it as my own experience, but this kind of imbalance happens across every sector of society. Many of us are trained from a young age to overwork, produce, and achieve at the expense of our health, rest, and relationships. This is the addiction no one really talks about. We can throw ourselves into work and not deal with personal issues. We can bury our heads in goals and strategies, and ignore the hardships or unresolved pain in our past. It's easier to use work, or the responsibilities we have as parents (if we have children), as an excuse not to be present or emotionally available to the people we love the most.

We can also have a devotion toward something good that in reality is bad, negative, or harmful for us. When out of moderation, our well-intended devotion can become destructive. We try to rationalize that we have everything under control. We can stop when we want to, right? After all, we have stopped drinking, smoking, overworking, or whatever it is, for periods of time in the past, so we can't be addicted, right? This is the beginning of the rationalizing we do when addiction is creeping up on us. We get confident when we are sober or abstain from our drug of choice for a period, and we even congratulate ourselves for having days when we are clean or don't use. Then we tell ourselves we can handle it when we partake again.

However, when we are falling into this rationalization of our behavior, even though it has negative consequences, we are falling into the trap of addiction. Remember, it is subtle until it is urgent. You must be killing your sin, or your sin will be killing you. Own your addiction before it owns you.

If you already feel like your addiction owns you, I wonder, Are you at rock bottom in your situation? That may not be a bad thing! J. K. Rowling said in a speech, "Rock bottom became the solid foundation on which I rebuilt my life."[5] This was true for me too. If

I had not hit rock bottom and gone to rehab, I don't know where I would be today. If you had told me that I would be healthy, happy, in a solid marriage, and living my best life, while helping people walk in freedom, I would not have believed it.

Overcoming Shame-Based Thinking by Reframing

In the new normal, there will be many "firsts." Every time you have a new first, you will also face what happened the last time you were in that same situation and have the opportunity to reframe it. You may still experience the familiar intense feelings of pain, shame, remorse, and grief; however, with new tools you can respond in a more effective and beneficial way. Learn to feel it, talk yourself through it, speak the truth, and let it go. You may even have an opportunity to make amends, say you are sorry, ask for forgiveness, and forgive yourself. We *get to* write the new story when we decide to reframe our distorted thinking.

Cognitive reframing is a technique used to shift your mindset so you're able to look at a situation, person, or relationship from a slightly different perspective. Cognitive reframing is something you can do at home or anytime you experience distorted thinking, but it can be helpful to have a therapist's assistance, particularly if you are caught in a negative thought pattern. When the technique is used in a therapeutic setting and practiced with the help of a therapist, it is known as cognitive restructuring.[6]

The essential idea behind reframing is that the frame through which a person views a situation determines their point of view. For example, for a long time when I thought about how I couldn't drink anymore, I felt like I was missing out. Over time, by practicing a new point of view in which I focus on the positive things I experience by not drinking, my thinking has shifted the meaning of what abstinence from alcohol means to me. No longer is it a bad thing not to drink. When the meaning changes, our thinking and behavior often change along with it. Eventually, my new perspective has become, *I get to not drink*, and that is exciting and inspiring and encouraging.

Work It Out

Step 11 is: "Sought through prayer and meditation to improve our conscious contact with God, as we understood Him, praying only for knowledge of His will for us and the power to carry that out." Our new normal requires regular, consistent check-ins with ourselves. Daily time spent with God in prayer, Bible reading, and examination of our hearts and thought lives creates the self-awareness we need to forge ahead in recovery.

We can ask God to show us daily what areas we need to address that we may be blinded to or unaware of. He can reveal to us why we are anxious, what pain or unforgiveness we are holding on to that is blocking us from intimacy and connection with Him. By habitually practicing this, we will find peace and harmony within ourselves. We are humbling ourselves and admitting our wrongs to God and people by making amends where necessary.

With our hearts clear, we can test our thoughts and reality-check them, holding on to what is true and letting go of the rest. As 1 Thessalonians 5:21 says, "Test everything; hold fast what is good" (ESV).

New Normal = Continual Surrender

Your new normal will require you to surrender continually. Step 11 requires us to surrender to God and give up our way of thinking that we can handle life and our recovery on our own. We must accept that we need God. When we don't truly surrender to a power greater than ourselves, we are in danger of doing life and recovery in our own strength, which we were never meant to do. We run out of strength, because we in our own flesh and humanity are limited beings. We can find comfort in God, for He is not limited in grace and power. He is sovereign and desires more than anything for us to receive His great love and tender mercies. We can receive all that He has to offer us when we surrender to Him, because He is faithful, and His love never ends. Psalm 107:1 says, "Give thanks to the LORD, for he is good; his love endures forever." Lamentations 3:22–23 says, "Because of the LORD's great love we are not consumed, for his compassions never fail. They are new every morning; great is your faithfulness."

I thank God for His great faithfulness to us when ours dwindles, fades, and drifts in our weakest moments. And that is such a great comfort to lean into on the road to recovery.

As much as we have a desire and every intention to make better choices, stay the course, stop the habit, and change our negative thought life, our own strength only gets us so far. Our flesh (humanity) is weak, and our strength will eventually wane. Spending time with God in prayer strengthens our spirit and connection to God, and it is the Spirit that gives us the strength to overcome temptation when we are weak. Jesus said in

> I thank God for His great faithfulness to us when ours dwindles, fades, and drifts in our weakest moments.

Matthew 26:41, "Keep watch and pray, so that you will not give in to temptation. For the spirit is willing, but the body is weak!" (NLT).

Finding a new normal also includes understanding the full impact of our addiction on the people in our lives, and that's what we'll explore next.

PART 3

Do the Work

A Framework for Getting Healthy and
Managing a Healthier Way of Life

CHAPTER 10

The Family Disease

At some point in our lives, we all say, "It will never happen to me!" Yet addiction is not a respecter of persons and can happen to anyone. A survey completed by Gallup in 2019 found that the effects of substance abuse are felt by around half of all American families. Only slight differences were recorded by the survey regarding race or sex. Forty-six percent of US adults reported having dealt with substance abuse in their families. Eighteen percent said those were related only to alcohol, while 10 percent said their problems were related only to drugs. Another 18 percent said they had dealt with both.[1]

Addiction is a family disease. Families are just as sick emotionally as the person in the addiction. They spend time, energy, prayer, emotion, money, and more trying desperately to help loved ones who are dealing with addictions. Families of addicts have many questions: *Is it my fault? What did I do or not do? What could I do to make them stop struggling? Why don't they just decide to stop? Don't they love me enough to stop?* Or maybe you have tried ignoring things, pretending they aren't happening, hoping they will go away. But they don't. It gets worse. You get more desperate for change. The big dream for a happy family is a fantasy that you watch others experience but seems unattainable for you. You find yourself grieving the relationship you wish you had with your loved one, and addiction makes it impossible to make that a reality.

We're raised watching our parents/caregivers, and we do what they do. We have to unlearn behaviors we pick up from childhood. Children of addicts fall into cycles of mistrust and silence. They pretend things are not as bad as they are or cover for the behaviors and outbursts of their parents, or even their neglect, out of shame. They walk around numb and disconnected—it's too risky to stay connected to their true emotions, because they fear falling apart if they allow themselves to feel. Children need security to grow into confident adults who are independent and wise decision makers. But with addiction as a constant presence, their childhood is full of insecurity, because they never know what to expect. Children of adults with substance-abuse issues often wonder when or if Mom or Dad will get sober; whether their parent will provide food and other basic needs for them; and if their parent will hurt them or fly off the handle and embarrass them. *Do they really love me?* they wonder.

Many children are forced to choose a side because their parents play tug-of-war with them, creating a depth of guilt that leaves them feeling powerless. The impact plays out into adulthood through the development of negative patterns of behavior, such as being overly responsible for their own lives or trying to control every outcome, feeling paralyzed, or being incapable of taking responsibility for their own lives. The adult child of an alcoholic can become dysfunctional in the sense that they live in extremes and either do too much or nothing at all to adjust to their ever-changing and uncertain lives.

The family needs to recover together whenever it is possible. Steps can be taken to address and break dysfunctional family systems that lead to continued cycles of addiction being passed down from one generation to the next. Jeremiah 32:18 says, "You show unfailing love to thousands, but you also bring the consequences of one generation's sin upon the next" (NLT). If we don't deal with generational cycles of dysfunction, our children will be left with the fallout of them.

When we don't talk about our experiences with the challenges we faced growing up, or inform children that there is clinical depression, bipolarity, autism, ADHD, or some other mental health issue or addiction in our families, then our offspring are left unaware. This lack of awareness has consequences of its own. Our children will experience challenges in their mental health with no backstory or family history to help them understand that they are susceptible to addiction or that they are not alone, crazy, or bad for their mental health issues. What if shame or stigma didn't keep us from sharing our family history? We'd stand a better chance of getting the help we need sooner and avoid severe consequences that addiction or undealt-with mental health issues may bring. Each generation has the choice to let their natural inclination repeat the negative cycle or find a better way.

Jimmy and I have decided that *it stops with us*! Our children will understand our family history of ADHD and how to handle it for themselves. They will understand symptoms of anxiety and depression, and not be afraid to ask for help. They won't have to wallow in shame and misery about mental health challenges they might face. I determined to share my experiences with addiction and how it crept up on me. Sharing the facts about the nature of addiction helps our kids make their own empowered choices. I can't force my kids not to drink just because I fear they will deal with alcoholism like I have. It's been hard to accept, but I have released that the decision belongs to them. My part as a parent is offering a safe place and resources to talk about the effects of addiction and mental health on a person. All I can do is lift the shame and stigma associated with addiction and mental health and pray that they make choices that benefit themselves.

Family Week at the Meadows

As angry as Jimmy was at me for still not admitting my problem with alcohol, he came out to family week at the Meadows rehab center. This is where we learned the importance of the family healing together. Let me walk you through some of the revelations we shared, with the hope that you might see yourself and your loved ones in our struggles and changes.

During family week, loved ones joined us for our recovery process. We were all learning about addiction, trauma, PTSD, and codependency and its effect on a person's brain and behaviors. This was a key turning point for Jimmy as he became aware of why and what brought us to this crisis point. Through the group counseling sessions, Jimmy said, "My wife is choosing alcohol over me and our kids. I feel like she is cheating on me with alcohol, and I am angry that she won't admit she has a problem." He believed that I could stop drinking if I just made the decision to do it. His anger and blame for the disaster of our relationship was centered around me, and he felt my drinking was personal toward him.

I remember Jimmy saying, "I can lead a church, but I can't lead my wife." He felt like he could pastor a church of thousands but could not talk to the one person he laid his head down on the pillow next to at night. He said, "I am successful and lead a thriving church with an incredible children's ministry, but why is it that my kids struggle to talk to me? How did we get so dysfunctional? This seems too far gone to fix. Maybe we shouldn't be married."

Our counselor said, "Jimmy, if you leave her, the new Irene won't have the opportunity to heal the wounds the old Irene created."

We cannot avoid being triggered, and Jimmy no longer wanted to feel the pain of constantly bracing himself for the disappointment that I would drink again and things would never change. The counselor urged him to learn to process through the trigger, face the fear, and take the risk that he may get disappointed if we were going to heal and save our marriage.

Jimmy asked her, "But what if it doesn't work?"

She answered him by saying, "But, Jimmy, what if it does? I understand your apprehension. This is normal and valid. Let's answer the 'what if' questions you have. What if Irene came home a different person and you also benefited from the process of recovery this crisis has forced on you? What if you used this crisis to benefit and grow your marriage rather than allow it to destroy your family?"

This all felt so mysterious and unbelievable to Jimmy. How would he know if the change in my behavior was real or if it was a performance? Was he willing to spend the rest of his life constantly bracing himself for impact of a relapse? It seemed too painful to hope for change that may just be temporary and leave him disappointed all over again. He was exhausted from the roller coaster of hope and disappointment he had been on for the past several years. As I listened to understand him rather than defend myself, I began to feel his pain and see things from his point of view. Something was beginning to shift in my perspective toward him. I began to see that underneath his anger was pain.

Jimmy shared in our counseling sessions (I am sharing with his permission, of course!) that he felt insecure, like there was something wrong with him because he felt I needed to drink to be with him intimately. This deep insecurity, and the wounds I caused during my blackouts (who knows what hurtful things I said or did, because I can't remember them) caused pain and resentment in his soul that fueled his anger toward me.

Through the mediation and counseling, I began to see Jimmy not as the angry husband, but as the person I injured. The person I vowed to love but hurt deeply, even if not deliberately. I learned compassion for him that I never had before, when I was also filled with resentment, blaming him for my misery. This compassion was reciprocated toward me in the sessions when he learned how PTSD is an injury to the brain. My triggers and behaviors were not personal toward him but came from experiences well before I met him. In our lack of awareness, he triggered my wounds, and I triggered his. We were stuck in a destructive cycle of hurt and pain, desperate to find a way out. The eye-opening experience of hearing, learning, and understanding each other's pain and experiences stopped the cycle right in its tracks. But that was just the beginning of the healing journey.

Acknowledgment of the Part We Play

Counselor: "Jimmy, do you realize that you were enabling
Irene's drinking?"

Jimmy: "What? There is no way! What do you mean I
am an enabler? I don't make her drink!"

If an enabler is a person or thing that makes something possible, or who encourages or enables negative or self-destructive behavior in another, then by definition Jimmy was an enabler. In his anger, he would send shaming messages to get me to stop drinking, but instead it drove me to drink more and hide my drinking. No, he did not make me drink, because no one can make us do anything. But he contributed to my addiction whenever he said it was okay for me to have a glass of wine with dinner or said yes to avoid an argument.

Jimmy realized he was just as sick emotionally as I was sick in my addiction. We both needed healing. We both needed recovery. We both needed to work to heal, and we both needed to make amends with each other. Again, addiction is a family disease, and approaching it from the standpoint that the loved ones of the addict are just as sick emotionally as the person in the addiction solidifies that we all need to recover together.

If you find yourself blaming others, making excuses, or lying to cover the addict's behavior, you are functioning as an enabler. Are you resenting the addict for their behaviors even though they are not themselves and the drug is controlling them? Do you avoid and ignore the negative behaviors and pretend they are not happening? Maybe you avoid bringing things up or arguing, anticipating that the addict will attempt to rationalize their behavior or manipulate you into thinking you are crazy. Acknowledging that we might be enabling a loved one in their addiction is tough, but it is a necessary step to healing.

Having compassion for someone's pain when they are causing us pain is difficult. The apostle Paul explained how we can go into someone else's world and experience it from their point of view with empathy and with the goal of understanding their perspective. We don't have to agree. We don't have to compromise our own standards or values. We want to send the message that we won't judge, but we won't excuse dysfunction either. Paul didn't just want to talk about it; he wanted to be in on it!

> Even though I am free of the demands and expectations of everyone, I have voluntarily become a servant to any and all in order to reach a wide range of people: religious, nonreligious, meticulous moralists, loose-living immoralists, the defeated, the demoralized—whoever. I didn't take on their way of life. I kept my bearings in Christ—but I entered their world and tried to experience things from their point of view. I've become just about every sort of servant there is in my attempts to lead those I meet into a God-saved life. I did all this because of the Message. I didn't just want to talk about it; I wanted to be *in* on it! (1 Corinthians 9:19–23 MSG)

Maybe it's time to see your struggling loved one in a different light. Perhaps they really can't stop without help and need you to be the safe place where they let down their guard and accept the help they truly need. Let's be in on the change we want to see in our families and our loved ones. We can't change them, but we can love them to a God-saved life through empathy, compassion, and understanding, and that love will potentially open the door for them to trust that we have their best interests in mind as we encourage them to get well.

Family Meetings

A tool that changed the trajectory of our marriage and family relationships is the family meeting. The Meadows treatment center taught this concept during family week to help families heal, and we were greatly impacted by it.[2] This tool helped us go from being dysfunctional to functional in our communication. Let me stop and say here that families look different for everyone. Not all of you are married with children. Using the concepts outlined in this tool helps resolve conflict in *any* relationship. Maybe right now your family consists of the roommates you live with, or perhaps you're a single parent rebuilding after loss. Maybe you are no longer close to your family of origin but have developed incredible friends who feel like family through a faith community. Whatever your family looks like as you heal, please know that you can adjust this tool to cultivate closeness, connection, and understanding among the family you love. This tool works for families who are ready to participate and willing to grow together.

The great news about this communication tool is that it will eventually impact all your other relationships by teaching you how to have meaningful communication that heals. The goal is to provide a safe place to share emotions without interruption and to promote the art of listening.

We found it was critical to establish clear guidelines for our family meetings so everyone was on the same page with how the boundaries would work. Doing so helped us create an environment that felt safe enough for us to be vulnerable. We learned to actively listen to understand rather than seek to respond. We chose a regular time to meet that was sacred: Wednesday evenings at 7:00 p.m. No one made plans, and all phones were off during this time. We took turns opening each meeting in prayer, then we reviewed our established ground rules. They looked like this:

- When one person talked, all others listened without judgment.
- Only the person with the "talking stick" (we used a baton, but you can use a remote, spoon, or whatever works) could talk. All others listened and avoided defensive body language or making fun of one another.
- The person sharing would pass the baton to indicate when they were finished.
- We would thank and acknowledge the person who'd shared before going to the next person.
- There was no interrupting or trying to fix or resolve any problems during this meeting time. Only questions for clarification could be asked. (Note that parents can follow up privately, after the meeting is over, with younger children on important issues that may arise.)
- We set a timer to keep shares between two and three minutes long, so short attention spans wouldn't drift.
- Each person took a turn owning their feelings using "I" statements about basic emotions (e.g., joy, love, anger, fear, etc.). For example, I would say, "I experienced joy this week when I went to AA and received a chip to celebrate ninety days of sobriety." I felt pain when my children expressed moments where they felt fear or pain when I was drinking. My husband

expressed that he felt anger when he found empty liquor bottles hidden around the house while I was gone at rehab. My daughter said, "I feel love when I see Mom work on her sobriety and her recovery, because I feel like she loves herself and loves our family."

So much healing happened in our family meetings as we listened to one another and became intimately acquainted with each other's emotions. The hardest part for me as a recovering codependent was trying not to fix the issues and instead leaning into the experience of the sharer with empathy. That is where our bond was sealed. Going into someone else's world and experiencing it from their point of view without judgment—whether we agreed with their emotion or not—helped us all feel heard.

Our conversations evolved into overall better communication, where we shared what we felt when we heard another person say something, or when we observed something in someone's behavior. For example, my son once said to my husband, "When I heard you yell at me and say my room was not clean enough, what I made up about that was that I would never do a good enough job for you. I felt sadness, shame, and anger." My husband was able to hear the felt need and address that in his response by acknowledging how Jaden felt first. My son took ownership over how he felt without criticizing the way his father acted, which made Jimmy receptive to hear what Jaden had to say.

Ultimately, when we felt acknowledged, we would process that what we were "feeling" wasn't necessarily the truth. And once our family members acknowledged our feelings, they could adjust their behaviors and be more mindful about their future communication. We had tremendous healing breakthrough in and out of our family meetings. With enough practice, the guidelines taught us how to have this type of safe, healing conversation in our daily interactions.

Here are two additional tips to help your family meetings succeed:

- Think of ways everyone can participate and look forward to the time together each week—things like family pizza night before the meeting, then family game time after the meeting. Promoting positive connection and interaction before and after the meeting will create positive memories around these family meetings and solidify that this new habit is a good one. The family will keep coming back because they will anticipate a time to be heard, seen, and connected as a family unit.

- Google "emotions charts" and paste these charts around the house to normalize the labeling and expressing of emotions. Normalizing emotions and learning to label them appropriately will be sure to change the dynamic in your family's communication and processing of emotions.

Learning transformative communication through family meetings brings healing. Learning to use new skills helps people listen, talk, and determine better talking and listening boundaries. When people feel heard, negativity in conflict is diffused, and the door to forgiveness and healing is opened. As a result of our healing, we are not only closer as a family but have greater health and influence in all our relationships. Take courage that something greater—immeasurably more amazing than you could have ever hoped for or dreamed—is on the other side of all the work. We can laugh with true joy and be present for ourselves to heal while being present for our families to heal and recover as well.

Projection

Projection is a defense mechanism people use to avoid feeling discomfort. This is important to talk about in relation to our loved ones, because connecting again, learning new ways of relating and healing together, is vulnerable work.

Licensed clinical social worker Karen Koenig has said, "Projection refers to unconsciously taking unwanted emotions or traits you don't like about yourself and attributing them to someone else."[3] Projecting looks different for everyone. For example, someone who won't stop talking accuses another person of not being a good listener when they cut off the talker just to get a word into the conversation. Or a cheating spouse becomes paranoid and accuses their partner of being unfaithful when it is really them who is cheating. Or an adult who was physically abused by their parents may act out in the very same way toward their own children after vowing they would never be like their parents.

In my case, I realized I dealt with rejection and abandonment issues from my childhood experiences, whether it was real from a bullying experience or a script I made up in my mind about my father leaving to go work overseas. I felt abandoned, unloved, not enough, and rejected by my dad, yet the reality was he had to go work to provide for our family. Deep down inside, I felt like I was never enough, and this led to the unconscious belief that Jimmy didn't want to be around me when he left home for a speaking engagement. What I made up wasn't true, yet I would defend myself from experiencing this pain by drinking to numb it, emotionally detaching myself from Jimmy. I remember after my father came home from being away for a year, rather than jumping into his arms to welcome him home, I extended my hand to greet him. I was a ten-year-old little girl who desperately missed her father. The handshake response did not line up with those emotions, but the detachment was a form of protection. I continued to repeat this kind of self-protection by using responses that did not match my true emotions and feelings into adulthood.

My work as an adult was to practice reversing these scenarios by becoming aware of my feelings and the temptation to numb them and protect myself. When the feeling of inadequacy or rejection came up, thanks to somatic therapy and recovery work, I was able to identify where I felt it in my body. Since our bodies are deeply attached to our emotions, we have physical responses to pain, fear, and vulnerability. I feel rejection and not being enough in my gut, and my work, as for all of us with traumatic backgrounds, is to acknowledge it. Listening to our bodies helps us become acutely aware of our triggers and the emotions we experience as a result.

The next step in recognizing when you are projecting is to "hold your space," as my counselor would say, visualizing a Plexiglas wall in front of you with a mirror. The Plexiglas represents the boundary, and you get to filter and decide what comes in as your truth. The mirror represents reflecting back what you hear and, in some cases, returning what doesn't belong to you to the person you are communicating with. I take the following steps to reality-check my thoughts, filter what I am hearing, and decide what to do with my thoughts as I respond, resolve, and move forward:

1. *Is this thought true?* I ask. When triggered, I get to decide if the trigger or what someone said about me is real or true.

2. I get curious. I ask, *Where is this coming from? Is there evidence or data that is for or against my thought? Am I worrying about something I can't control?* I can detach from myself by holding my space and then getting curious about what I am experiencing without judgment. I ask myself exploratory questions, like, *Is this 100 percent true about me?*

3. Then I consider, *How do I feel about this thought?* I notice story lines that I am holding on to and name my feelings or emotions about them. I may feel angry, jealous, or hurt. Labeling our emotions is a powerful tool.

4. I question, *What if I looked at things differently, from a positive standpoint? Can I be generous and believe the best about this person by giving them the benefit of the doubt? Will their words matter a year from now? Is this thought helpful or causing me stress?* I imagine the benefits of a perspective shift to the relationship and picture a different outcome. I may even ask a trusted person who can be objective and rational what they think about my response.

Taking these steps will empower you to decide how you will move forward in a healthy way. You can reflect or mirror back what you are hearing to the person speaking. You can be honest and communicate about how you feel or what you are experiencing by owning what you are feeling. Rather than projecting issues that belong to you, you can own your reality and not put it on someone else.

In my dysfunction, I would project my feelings about myself onto my family and avoid them altogether, which hurt them. Or I would shut down or hide my true self from them to protect myself. The new outcome was freeing when I began to square my shoulders and own my power of defining how I was going to feel about myself. The healed Irene knows I am enough because God says I am enough. The healed Irene intuitively knows that the verbal darts being thrown really don't have anything to do with me, but with the person throwing them. My work is to practice holding space without taking personally what the person is saying and be courageous enough to share my experience and reflect back what I'm hearing. Most times, once I communicate what I am hearing, I am able to sort through what is real and what is a script and land on a healthy thought moving forward.

We must take extreme ownership of and responsibility for our own wounds. Not false responsibility, where we try to fix something that doesn't belong to us or isn't ours to fix, but responsibility for our part. This is tough in families with codependent dynamics. Personally, I wanted to make amends and own *my part* with my family without them feeling like I was being codependent, trying to cover or excuse Jimmy's infractions and poor behavior that also hurt and created fractures in the family dynamic. I realized I had to apologize for my part and leave it at that. Not trying to fix it all was part of my healing from codependency. Each member of the family has a process to own, and I had to let go of trying to be the fixer.

Over time my family had to see the change in us for themselves and reconcile how they would feel about us moving forward. After all, I was responsible for oversharing in my drunken vents to my sisters and brothers, which had created the relational triangle with Jimmy and me on opposing ends and my family at the

> We must take extreme ownership of and responsibility for our own wounds.

other. This caused pain and division within all parties involved. I imagine they wondered if we had really changed or if they were seeing a performance. The saying goes that time heals all wounds, and it would take my letting go of what reconciliation would look like and accepting that I could only do my part, which was to ask for forgiveness and give them space to process. Just as I had to hold my space, my new perspective of exercising healthy boundaries required me to allow them to do the same.

Developing Healthy Relationships

You may be wondering if it is possible to develop healthy relationships when you feel like they have been nothing but dysfunctional all your life. Yes, it is possible, but it takes more than wishing for them. Becoming aware of dysfunction and how you have operated in it, then finding tools to flip the script and develop healthier relationships, is as possible for you as it has been for me.

You might be surprised by how well your loved ones take on the healthy tools you demonstrate and desire the change and freedom they see in you. Initially, they may not like when you operate in new healthier patterns, because dysfunction in families feels familiar, and that makes people feel secure. Change sometimes freaks out people, and they don't always know what to do with it. That's okay. There will always be those people who prefer the dysfunctional you and will attempt to keep you as that person. They may test you to see if the change is real. They have always been able to count on the dysfunction, and fear of change can make them feel like they are losing control. It will take time, communication, and consistency to break unhealthy patterns and to bear fruit, so they can see that they, too, can benefit and have mutually satisfying relationships.

What You Can Do

Many ask me, as I travel for speaking events, about how to help someone who they're noticing is slipping into addiction. This may sound cliché, but prayer is always key as a first response rather than a last resort. Prayer has power to change hearts. Only God knows a person's heart and intentions, and the Holy Spirit can give you wisdom, grace, and courage to have hard conversations. We are not able to do what God can do, and sometimes our history with the person hinders or complicates their ability to hear from us. As you pray, if you sense an invitation to speak to them, communicate and be honest with your loved one in a kind and nonjudgmental way. Explain what you notice without accusation. Share concern and empathy and ask how you can help and if they are open to getting help. Sometimes creating that safe place for the person to be heard can make all the difference in their acceptance of help. I know it's hard to leave the rest of the intervention to God to take care of, but releasing the responsibility of your loved one to God frees you!

Getting educated about addiction and how you can help yourself and your loved one who is struggling with addiction is critical, along with being part of a family support group like Celebrate Recovery, Al-Anon, Alateen, or others. These family support groups can help families and friends of alcoholics find hope, healing, and encouragement through shared experiences, information, and connection in meetings. Too often we focus on the person we view as sick in the addiction. Maybe it's time we flip the script and help ourselves first. Together we grow and together we heal the family disease of addiction and codependency. May the Serenity Prayer bring you peace in the days ahead.

> God grant me the serenity
> To accept the things I cannot change,
> Courage to change the things I can,
> And wisdom to know the difference.

CHAPTER 11

Holistic Healing

O ur bodies hold our stories, our memories, and our experiences. We cannot divorce the body from the head and the heart. Our recovery must be holistic, addressing the physical (including mental health), spiritual, emotional, and medical aspects of our lives. We must incorporate body, mind, and soul in our recovery. Many people ignore the holistic connection between these three parts and get stuck—struggling to overcome. I understand why! Recovery in all these areas is not only a lot of work, but it takes a lot of time.

I did a lot of therapy prior to going to rehab, but it wasn't as effective because I was still drinking. As I mentioned earlier, my codependency issues were identified but not treated by my therapists. Rehab therapy was different because the holistic approach to my recovery included body, mind, and soul work in therapy as well as classes that gave me the "why" behind the "what" I was recovering from. This approach gave far better results. Equine therapy, yoga, tai chi, regular exercise, acupuncture, low-sugar diet, half-caffeinated/half-decaffeinated coffee? Hello?! I need my caffeine in the morning and midafternoon. And this was a long list of stuff to do! What I didn't realize when I entered rehab but learned over those forty days was how much these components were critical to the holistic nature of my recovery. I added these to my weekly rhythm, alongside talk therapy, AA meetings, Co-Dependents Anonymous meetings, Eye Movement Desensitization and Reprocessing (EMDR) therapy, group counseling, and even intense outpatient treatment. It was also important for me to learn to have fun, spend time in the morning praying and reading the Bible, practice mindfulness and meditation, and learn to be quiet and enjoy being alone. Rehab also gave me the opportunity to attend classes to learn about the brain, trauma, addiction, family dysfunction, healing the child within, codependency, and how all these things relate to the addictive cycle.

Expressing our feelings and emotions on a regular basis is an effective way to release pent-up trauma, pain, and negativity. Just speaking the truth out loud causes lies to lose their power. We release trauma and painful emotions when we practice grounding, discharging emotions in counseling or in a small group. The goal is to release the stress that is blocking us from truly relaxing. Following are various methods and tools to help you care for your whole person.

Physical ways to discharge stress and trauma are things like tai chi and yoga, in which we practice breathing and connection with our bodies. I like to think that yoga mimics recovery in the sense that it is painful and requires you to breathe. In recovery we must push through pain, take deep breaths, and get in touch with our bodies in order to heal, calm, and push through difficulty. Acupuncture and massage therapy are other methods that help relax our physical bodies and relax our nervous systems.

Practicing presence can be done through *mindfulness and meditation*. We are often distracted, hurried, and anxious. Learning to stay present in the moment helps calm the mind and body to resist the hurry and worry. Mayo Clinic defines mindfulness as "a type of meditation in which you focus on being intensely aware of what you're sensing and feeling in the moment, without interpretation or judgment. Practicing mindfulness involves breathing methods, guided imagery, and other practices to relax the body and mind and help reduce stress."[1]

Mindfulness and meditation are scientifically proven to improve our mental health and various conditions including stress, anxiety, pain, depression, insomnia, high blood pressure (hypertension), asthma, fibromyalgia, short attention spans, job burnout, sleep, and diabetes.[2]

Grounding oneself helps us to be present in the moment and is the process of balancing our physical, emotional, mental, and energy states and reconnecting them. We do this through allowing the bottoms of our feet or palms of our hands to connect with the earth. For me, my favorite is grounding on a beach and noticing what the sand feels like in my hands and under my feet. I appreciate life and the earth God created, and this centers me.

Michelle McDonald coined the RAIN acronym over twenty years ago as an easy-to-remember tool for developing mindfulness and awareness of oneself.

R—"Recognize what is going on."
A—"Allow the experience to be there, just as it is."
I—"Investigate with kindness."
N—"Natural awareness, which comes from not identifying
    with the experience."[3]

Fun is essential in developing the positive attitude needed to keep moving forward in recovery. All work and no play does not lead to balance but instead can contribute to feelings of dread, fatigue, and negativity. You may need to do some experimenting to rediscover what types of recreation refresh and revive you.

I have discovered that I love to read psychological thrillers for fun and to work out with my bootcamp class. Bootcamp class has become a nonnegotiable on my schedule for one hour three times a week. There I connect with other people and get challenged physically to push myself past my mental limitations. Yes, I find this fun. Not only do the endorphins help me feel better overall, but the camaraderie is food for my soul. A bonus is the boost to my self-esteem. I feel great in my jeans! I call this a nonnegotiable because when I don't work out, I notice that my mood changes, my ability to handle stress is challenged, and I find myself fighting anxiety. Working out is my medicine and a critical part of my investment in myself through recreation.

Group support is critical in recovery. We need people and we need God! All kinds of support groups are available—for grief, sex addiction, post-divorce care, love addiction, and more. Recovering alone is impossible. But there is something powerful and comforting about knowing that someone else has "been there and done that" and has experienced what we are going through. That helps us remember that we are not alone in our struggles. Most comforting of all, God promises never to leave us or forsake us (Deuteronomy 31:6), and He is with us through the fire and storms of life, holding us up and strengthening us (Isaiah 41:10). Take comfort that you are not alone.

When we stop learning, we stop growing. Reading books, articles, blogs, and the Bible helps keep your brain engaged, growing, and learning. Journaling is also therapeutic. I used journaling prompts in my recovery to help me get into the practice of checking in regularly, remembering to connect and care for myself so that I could reprogram the way I disconnected and disregarded myself in the past. Prompts can be as simple as these:

- Today I feel . . .
- Today I'm thankful for . . .
- God, I feel resentment about _____ and fear about _____. Please forgive me and remove this resentment and fear.
- God, please help me . . .

Overall health and wellness inform our mental and emotional state. This is not about dieting, but about loving yourself enough to nourish yourself with rest, body movement, hydration, and nutritious foods. You would be surprised how regular exercise or taking a walk and enjoying nature, eating healthy and hydrating, and decreasing your sugar or caffeine intake can make a difference in how you feel overall. Our bodies function so much better in homeostasis, or a state of balance.

The cafeteria in my rehab facility only offered half-caffeinated coffee, and sugar packets had to be requested from the line cook. Initially, I thought this was crazy because I felt I needed my sugar and my coffee to survive. But as I detoxed from alcohol, sugar, and caffeine, my body was able to get to a place of baseline function to rebuild from. Taking away all the extra junk my body was working hard to process gave me the ability to find a baseline in my body that my doctors could then build a treatment plan around to give my body what it needed to function effectively. I felt amazing! My skin looked amazing! And my mind was clear as I processed difficult things in recovery.

Reframe the Shame of Mental Health

Just as recovery gets a bad rap, so does mental health. Having a mental health struggle—whether a societal stigma or a family issue—is associated with shame. Mental health is too often disregarded or misunderstood, and many people lack awareness of how common mental health issues are.

Mental illnesses are among the most common health conditions in the United States. According to the Centers for Disease Control and Prevention, they affect more than 50 percent of Americans at some point during their lifetimes—including one in five children. What's more: "Mental health includes our emotional, psychological, and social well-being. It affects how we think, feel, and act. It also helps determine how we handle stress, relate to others, and make healthy choices" through every stage of our lives.[4]

Our mental health is where the brain comes into our recovery, and this is significant because the brain literally affects everything we do! Are you aware of any mental health challenges you may have, such as ADHD, ADD, bipolar disorder, generalized anxiety disorder, or depression, that are going unaddressed and making your life unmanageable? My entire family has been diagnosed with ADHD or ADD, and in our experience, this has been freeing because now we can address our lives with understanding of what we need to help us be our best selves. Some of us need medication for our executive function to be optimized, while others use natural remedies and cognitive behavioral therapy to improve our executive function. As a result, we are experiencing less anxiety because of the understanding about how our brains function. This plays out in everyday life as increased productivity, less procrastination, confidence in our learning, and ability to see projects and tasks through from start to finish. Unaddressed, our mental health issues can lead to unmanageable lives that can cause hopelessness and misery. If you are unsure about therapy, perhaps you are still dealing with stigmas associated with mental health. You deserve to be happy. Therapy is a proven way to get the help or diagnosis you need for your underlying mental health challenges, whether they are emotional or chemical related. I share more about some of the types of therapy and treatment options available below.

Counseling and Types of Therapy

Therapy has been a game changer for me, my marriage, and my family as we have healed together. If all the types of therapy are boggling your mind and you don't know where to start, the internet is your friend! Search and find out more about the different types of therapy available. Find a local licensed therapist or counselor to assist you on your recovery journey. If finances are an issue or you do not have medical insurance, many clinics and counseling centers have sliding scales for payment. There are also many low-cost virtual options for therapy. Here are a few types of therapy to consider:

- Eye Movement Desensitization and Reprocessing (EMDR) is a psychotherapy that enables people to heal from the symptoms and emotional distress that are the result of disturbing life experiences.[5]

- Somatic Experiencing (SE) therapy aims to treat the effects of PTSD and other mental and emotional health issues through the connection of mind and body, and uses a body-centric approach. This therapy helps to release physical stress, tension, and trauma, rather than only resolving problems verbally.[6]
- Emotion-Focused Therapy (EFT) is a therapeutic approach based on the premise that emotions are key to identity. According to EFT, emotions are a guide for individual choice and decision-making. This type of therapy assumes that lacking emotional awareness or avoiding unpleasant emotions can cause harm.[7]
- Imago Therapy or Imago Relationship Therapy (IRT) is a specific style of relationship therapy designed to help conflicts within relationships become opportunities for healing and growth. The term *imago* is Latin for "image," and within the context of IRT it refers to an "unconscious image of familiar love."[8]

Counseling Centers

Taking a time-out to retreat from the craziness of life and focus on reviving and restoring your soul, mind, and body is one of the best gifts you can give yourself. CrossRoads Counseling of the Rockies is a great place to go for a counseling retreat, whether you need it as an individual or for your entire family as a group. They also provide incredible marriage counseling (crisis and/or maintenance or reboot) and pastoral reboots, which my husband and I have taken advantage of over the course of our marriage. According to their website, they promote "both emotional and spiritual growth by integrating biblical principles with evidence-based treatment methods." The format used provides in-depth understanding of your problems, as well as tools to continue dealing with them at home.[9]

Treatment Centers – Outpatient vs. Inpatient

Finding a good treatment center is key. Not all treatment centers are meant to work for everyone because everyone's needs for recovery are different. I suggest working with a counselor or someone in your accountability circle and speaking with the intake specialists at various treatment centers to determine which program is a good fit for you. Research is everything!

Keep in mind that dual diagnosis is typically what many of us have going on. The addiction may just be a symptom of something else. Many of my friends in rehab ended up coming to The Meadows after a thirty-day stint in a detox medical rehab facility. Many of them had the same story—they went to a rehab facility to detox, then returned home only to relapse almost within days if not hours of returning home because the root issue of why they were using was not dealt with. Treatment centers like the one I went to at The Meadows treat dual diagnoses and cover other issues outside of addiction. I like to describe The Meadows as a healing center that treats addiction through the lens of trauma. Another option is to get detoxed and then perhaps find a local intensive outpatient program (IOP) and couple that with the type of counseling or therapy you need.

Workshops are another way to invest in yourself for growth

and recovery from any situation—trauma, relationship issues, codependency, inner-child healing, marriage problems, and so on. Many counseling centers offer such programs at a cost for a day or two or even up to a week or two. Participation in such workshops doesn't have to be all or nothing. Many options are available, including online options if you are unable to physically attend a workshop.

Outpatient Treatment Centers

Intense outpatient programs in your area may be an option. Most insurances cover the cost, and they offer individualized treatment planning, including but not limited to these:

- group therapy
- medication-assisted treatment
- detox when needed
- continuing care
- relapse prevention

The accountability of random drug and alcohol testing is also a benefit of these programs, to help in the sobriety journey. Outpatient centers typically offer 12-step program support groups such as AA, Narcotics Anonymous (NA), Al-Anon, and more. For people seeking treatment for alcohol or drug addiction, IOPs combine the effectiveness of inpatient treatment with the flexibility and affordability of outpatient care.

Inpatient Treatment Centers

Inpatient treatment can be critical for anyone dealing with any addiction, mental health issues, or trauma/PTSD (dual diagnosis).

There are specialized treatment locations for eating disorders, young adult treatment, sex addiction, and so on. Many also offer workshops to meet the needs of those who want enrichment in their recovery and healing, whether individuals, families, or couples.

A Series of Daily Decisions

As you can see, there are many ways to find help on your journey. Recovery is an uphill climb that begins with the decision to step out of denial and into reality. While it is freeing to accept the truth about where we are, it is also terrifying and painful. Whenever we decide to step out of hiding and into the unfamiliar place of honesty and vulnerability, we need to prepare ourselves to experience wonderful moments of freedom and difficult moments of endurance. It starts with a series of daily decisions. What is the next best thing you need to do to take care of yourself? It could be getting a massage, having quiet time with God, scheduling a therapy appointment, journaling, exercising, going to a support group meeting, reaching out to someone when you feel like your thought life is out of control and you feel crazy, or even just doing something fun.

My first ninety days after my last drink were fragile. Rehab opened me up to embrace life without alcohol, to wake up and make a series of daily, seemingly small and ordinary decisions, and to create new habits with large impact. One healthy coping mechanism applied repeatedly will become permanent over time. One day at a time, one hour at a time, one moment at a time—if you have to break it down to that level, you can do better for yourself and get free.

The key to living your best life can be found in making a series of small decisions, not just big ones. In fact, the more integrity we have in little things, the easier it is to make a big decision that lines up with our convictions and values. Sometimes we wait and pray and hope for a miracle to spontaneously be free from all our dysfunction, negative desires, and addictions—and I have known many people who have experienced such miracles from God. However, even after a spontaneous healing, there must be a process of renewing the mind that takes time.

Renewal

As Christians we are taught to speak the Word of God (the Bible) over ourselves when we feel weak and are struggling. I can testify that this most definitely works to ease into the Father's love and truth when I am emotionally overloaded. However, I don't believe we can act like just saying a scripture cures all our anxieties. Sure, there is a faith component; however, our bodies unforgivingly keep score of the trauma and stress we experience. Our bodies manifest this through anxiety and panic attacks, and many of us don't have the skills or awareness that these things must be dealt with and released. Stuffing, ignoring, and detaching doesn't work.

> The key to living your best life can be found in making a series of small decisions, not just big ones.

Neither does spiritualizing our pain and trauma and pretending like speaking Scripture over our situation will heal it all.

God is a fan of the process and of the renewing of the mind described in Romans 12. The apostle Paul wrote, "Don't copy the behavior and customs of this world, but let God transform you into a new person by changing the way you think. Then you will learn to know God's will for you, which is good and pleasing and perfect" (Romans 12:2 NLT). Renewal is a process of being made new again. After walking you through many options for a more holistic healing experience, it is also important for me to talk about our spiritual life and connection with God. Healing is a spiritual journey, which is why programs of recovery suggest finding God, or a "higher power," to pull strength from to walk out our recovery. My power and strength to walk out my recovery is found in my faith in Jesus Christ as my Lord and Savior. It is because of my personal relationship with Jesus and the faith I have in the Bible as my source for wisdom and life guidance that I am able to face the challenges of the recovery process. This is why I am able to accept the peace and grace I need to lead a happier and more fulfilling life of spiritual connectedness.

Where has your spiritual walk been interrupted or become stagnant and in need of a fresh start? What have you ignored that might be impacting your capacity to connect or your ability to change? Are you stuck in anger toward God, asking, *Why would God allow bad things to happen to me if He loves me?*

Why Church?

Maybe the whole church idea is a nonstarter for you because of scandals you have seen in the church, politics that turned you off. Or perhaps the racism issues or what is being said or not being said by church leaders has left a bad taste in your mouth. Maybe after the COVID-19 pandemic hit, you just never went back because you can attend church online, without having to connect with people.

The struggle is real because we need community to thrive, yet we don't want to go to church anymore. The news and reports we hear about church can be discouraging and fuel our mistrust in pastors, leaders, and quite frankly, the people in the pews!

Churches are full of hurting people, and sometimes hurt people hurt other people. The reality that our leaders are not perfect and struggle with real human conditions of the heart is fact. Are you able to consider that God can still use broken people to lead others spiritually, to help people in congregations learn to love the way Jesus did, and accept that we don't get it right all the time?

This is never an excuse for poor behavior from leaders or for people hurting other people; however, the reality is that we all are broken and need to walk out our salvation and spiritual growth. The whole purpose of coming to church to worship God is to connect with a power greater than ourselves. Hebrews 10:25 reminds us that we should not neglect meeting together. We need each other and we need God if we are going to get through the difficulties of life. Remember that 1 Thessalonians 5:20–21 says, "Test everything that is said. Hold on to what is good" (NLT). We can decide if we are connected to a healthy church. Look for signs of health, not perfection, because healthy things grow! Including you, if you're connected in a place that is life giving and serving people, where the leaders are humble before God.

I became disillusioned in my faith. Full of doubts and fears, I dealt with trust issues because of the pain that people in the church community caused me. We hear often about pastors hurting people, and that's real. Healthy accountability is needed for leaders who abuse power. But we do not often hear about the pain of the people hurting pastors. There are hurting people who hurt pastors who don't abuse their power. This particular pain piled onto the abuse from my past, my need to pretend and perform in order to be loved, and the shame I felt over having problems in the first place. I didn't know how to be honest or ask direct questions or engage in difficult conversations. What I came to realize through my journey of rediscovering God was that it would require a process of renewing my mind through the Word of God (the Bible) to unpack these questions, be vulnerable before God with them, and wait to find the answers I needed to progress forward and get unstuck.

Just as we have to search for a counselor who suits us, we need to find a church that feels right for us. Churches take on the personalities of their lead pastors, so you have to put in the same time and effort as you would seeking out a counselor to find a church where you can grow in your faith with others and build community. Being aware of where you are on the spectrum of self-care is important so you can address your needs—mind, body, and spirit.

We can be transformed, renewed, and restored if we are willing to do the work and submit to the process of renewing our minds and our relationship with God. We can't give up on the process of God doing something new in us. Second Corinthians 4:16 promises that if we don't give up, we will be renewed: "We do not lose heart. Though our outer self is wasting away, our inner self is being renewed day by day" (ESV).

I have come to find out that this process of renewal never ends. It is a continuum. We get stuck in cycles of doubt and fear because we worry that sharing our struggle with our faith, even as Christian leaders, would appear as weakness or hypocrisy. Yet we overcome by acknowledging our sin and brokenness and ultimately accepting the grace of God, who finds us, loves us, and doesn't give up on us.

The Promises of AA

If we are painstaking about this phase of our development, we will be amazed before we are halfway through. We are going to know a new freedom and a new happiness. We will not regret the past nor wish to shut the door on it. We will comprehend the word serenity and we will know peace. No matter how far down the scale we have gone, we will see how our experience can benefit others. That feeling of uselessness and self-pity will disappear. We will lose interest in selfish things and gain interest in our fellows. Self-seeking will slip away. Our whole attitude and outlook upon life will change. Fear of people and economic insecurity will leave us. We will intuitively know how to handle situations which used to baffle us. We will suddenly realize that God is doing for us what we could not do for ourselves.

Are these extravagant promises? We think not. They are being fulfilled among us—sometimes quickly, sometimes slowly. They will always materialize if we work for them.[10]

My favorite part of an AA meeting is when we read the Promises of AA. The shame of addiction and the negative patterns of thinking begin to come undone when we work our program of recovery and invite God into it. Our whole outlook on life changes as we develop a new pattern of thinking and behaving. There is something to the intentionality of repeating the same thing over and over each time we meet. The structure and repetition retrain the brain, and this is the renewing of the mind spoken about in Romans 12:2. We are reminded of the boundaries to adhere to at the beginning of each meeting, such as "Who you see here and what you say here, stays here." The confidentiality and anonymity provide a safe place for those like me who are suffering from toxic shame and full of fear, to make an effort to come out of our shells. There is no cross-talk at meetings, meaning we keep what we share to our own experience, and we do not try to fix someone else or comment on their share with our opinions, again creating a safe place for attendees to open up. Of course, people are human and broken, so there are some boundary violators; however, the "old-timers" (those with more than ten years of sobriety) are sure to address violations and bring things back into order.

The words *freedom, happiness, peace, serenity,* and *being a benefit to others* in the Promises have come true for me, and they can for you too! Not only that, but when we work our program of recovery, we will change our relationship with fear, regret, feelings of uselessness, self-pity, selfishness, and self-seeking that are par for the course when we are in an addiction.

Relapse Prevention

I remember hearing the term *pink elephant* in an AA meeting. I leaned over and asked the person next to me what that meant, and she explained drunken hallucinations. I was intimidated by all the recovery lingo and many times had to ask someone for understanding. Recovery felt almost like being in a secret society with its own language. About a year into my sobriety, I heard a warning come by way of an old-timer who shared at a Monday night meeting of my women's AA group.

She referred to a time that she was going through the motions of everything she "should do" after coming out of rehab. She eventually stopped going to meetings because she felt like she had done enough, and besides, she had removed alcohol from the equation, so she should be okay, right? Through her tears, she described how she became a "dry drunk" before she relapsed. She described the symptoms of being a dry drunk. She began to fantasize about her past drinking days and to ignore the negative consequences alcohol caused in her life. Mood swings became more frequent, and she found herself depressed and anxious, entertaining other unhealthy behaviors to cope. She spoke of falling into a victim mentality and negative thought patterns. Relapse was inevitable when she was home alone for a weekend and got a flu virus. When our physical bodies are compromised, our emotional world weakens, and we are more susceptible to making poor choices. It's when we are hungry, angry, lonely, or tired (HALT) that we are in danger of relapse. Being lonely, sick, tired, and at an emotional low, she found herself picking up the bottle again.

But this pattern doesn't apply just to alcoholism. Fill in the blank with whatever issue in which you are struggling not to relapse. My husband struggles with using food as his go-to, so relapse looks different for him. After emotionally taxing events or stress, he has the propensity to want to eat. He has described that he feels the compulsion to eat—eat a lot—and it has to be something he is craving in the moment if it's going to satisfy him. I support him by planning for those moments by having nutritional food available that tastes good. Jimmy also has to own his part of the struggle and work through making a decision to *eat to live, not live to eat*, while addressing the emotions he is feeling in the moment and not allowing them to drive his eating. Recovery is all about a series of decisions. When in doubt, just do the next right thing for yourself.

I felt the experience of the woman sharing in AA about her relapse and the pain and shame that came along with it as if it were my own. The thought of relapse scared me half to death. I had spent the past year celebrating every month with a new coin. Each time I brought one home, my husband and children would genuinely celebrate and congratulate me for another month of sobriety. Each time we celebrated a month, I felt so good about myself and the hard work I had done. The annual celebrations of my sobriety are even better than my birthday! My family goes all out. I like to call my yearly "sober-versaries" my "re-birthdays." The thought of relapsing and disappointing my family, hurting them all over again, and the shame of having to pick up another twenty-four-hour chip and start all over is enough to make me run from the sight of alcohol! Celebrate each win like you are receiving a reward for your next best choice! Celebrate when you put the laptop or phone away and choose to do something else besides watching porn. It's okay to give yourself a pat on the back and share your win with your accountability friends each time you say no to something the old codependent you would have said yes to.

This woman had done so much work, wasn't drinking, and thought she was good, but she fell right back into negative patterns that led to relapse. People who white-knuckle it and stop drinking on their own are at risk of becoming dry drunks and are at higher risk for relapse. The importance of working not only on not drinking but also on exploring why you drank or used and what led up to your using in the first place is a critical part of the recovery journey and relapse prevention. It's important to have a support group, counselor, or accountability partner you can be honest with to help identify and work through why you behave like or crave what you do.

My biggest takeaway from the woman's share is the warning that if we do not seek treatment for the underlying issues or psychological drivers of our addiction, we are at risk for relapse. There's a good chance we will continue to deal with and suffer from significant mental and emotional pain and turmoil even in the absence of our drug of choice. This not only leads to a lack of wholeness and happiness but also increases the potential of relapse. Note to self: *If you are not working on your recovery, you are working on relapse.* All I knew is that I did not want to become a dry drunk—a shell of a person exhibiting the same behaviors as when I was sick in my addiction, except without the substance. I decided that this was not going to be my story and I was going to learn from her pain so I didn't have to create any more for myself. To remain sober, recovery and sobriety must be the number one thing I commit to. I want more for you than just the end of substance abuse or addiction. Freedom from the pain, turmoil, dysfunction, and trauma is possible for you.

> If you are not working on your recovery, you are working on relapse.

And like they say in the church, if you are in agreement, "Can I get a good amen?"

CHAPTER 12

Reframe Your Shame

Michelle Graham wrote, "Shame says because I am flawed, I am unacceptable. Grace says because I am flawed, I am cherished."[1] Too often we believe that if we are vulnerable, it will be the end of us. We fear that if we are brave enough to touch the pain buried underneath the ways we hide, it might ruin our relationships and reputation. Shame keeps us overwhelmed and afraid of reaching out and sharing the truth of our story. Friend, if you don't know by now, it is all a lie. The truth is this: you can be free.

Allowing people to see the real me was not the end of me but the beginning of God doing something *new* in me. Letting people into my addiction and my mess of a life produced healing in my mind, body, and soul. Learning how to say, "I need help!" got me the empathy, acceptance, grace, and forgiveness that I needed to change. Today I am a living, breathing, walking, talking testimony of God's miracle-working redemptive power.

Shame was a sickness hidden deep in my soul that kept me

from engaging in life socially with people I didn't know, and it even showed up with people I love. I couldn't connect authentically while automatic thoughts popped up in my mind that said, *I don't deserve nice things or good things to happen to me, I don't deserve to be noticed or loved.* I kept my head down, avoiding eye contact and making excuses that I was just a shy person. The truth is I am far from shy, and one of my strengths is connection. Not only do I long for it, but I am good at connecting with people. I don't spend all my time and energy hiding now; rather, I find myself connecting and relating in an authentic way with other people. I find myself being truly known and accepted with my flaws and all, which has been a desire of my heart all along. I have finally accepted that God loves me just as I am! That I am enough because God says I am enough. I am inherently worthy. God's grace is sufficient for me. His grace gives me the strength I need to continue to walk out my recovery, share my story, and kick shame in the face! I own my story. I own my work. I own this messy yet beautiful process of recovery, self-discovery, and forgiveness of myself and others, and I want that more than anything for you as well. I embrace the *new* creation that I am. Through a process of renewal, the old is gone. I don't regret my past, because it made me who I am today. Second Corinthians 5:17 says, "If anyone is in Christ, the new creation has come: The old has gone, the new is here!"

Isaiah 43:18–20 (NLT) says:

> But forget all that—
>   it is nothing compared to what I am going
>   to do.
> For I am about to do something new.
>   See, I have already begun! Do you not see it?

I will make a pathway through the wilderness.
    I will create rivers in the dry wasteland.
The wild animals in the fields will thank me,
      the jackals and owls, too,
        for giving them water in the desert.
Yes, I will make rivers in the dry wasteland
      so my chosen people can be refreshed.

Neural pathways are created in our brains through repetition in our behaviors and habits. Simply put, it is as if we have deep grooves or roads in our brain. Just because we have formed these neural pathways doesn't mean they have to stay that way forever. Through repetition of new behaviors and ways of thinking, we can create a new normal, a new road, a new way of life.[2] In the process, you will be refreshed. Anything in your life that you experienced shame about can be *reframed*. New and healthy ways of doing life are available to you if you are willing to do the work. The Holy Spirit is already at work in you—can you begin to see it? He is opening your eyes to things you were unaware of before reading this book.

God is the great author of all our stories! Hebrews 12:2 says that Jesus is "the author and finisher of our faith" (NKJV). He is not done writing my story, and He is not done writing yours either! You can reclaim the power of what has been holding you back and reframe your shame.

Flawsome: (adj.) "the state of embracing one's flaws and knowing that one is awesome regardless"

My counselor gave me the homework assignment to look at myself in the mirror and affirm myself. This was awkward! I forced myself to look into my own eyes and tell myself, "You are beautiful, you are loved, you are enough, God loves you, you are worthy of love, you belong." Slowly, over time while repeating this exercise, what I saw in the mirror began to change. I saw myself for what seemed like the first time. I noticed my scars, freckles, and imperfections, and I repeated scripture to myself, saying, "I am fearfully and wonderfully made by God. I was made in the secret place, and nothing is hidden from God" (Psalm 139:14–15, my paraphrase). Before long, I began to accept who I was—scars, flaws, and all. My scars have made me beautiful.

Being me is finally satisfying. No more striving. I accept and love my flaws because I know I am awesome regardless! I am *flawsome*! I adopted this term after realizing that perfectionism was not serving me well. Recovery has taught me to embrace my imperfections, brokenness, and humanity. It's crazy how I love my body more today than ever, stretch marks and all. Just as pregnancy stretched me when I carried my babies, recovery stretched me and left scars that I now see as beautiful because of what that stretching produced. I don't have to mask or cover up my flaws, or hide them behind superficial things like performance, perfection, achievement, or anyone else's idea of success. I can be totally vulnerable, free to be myself, because God loves me just the way I am and accepts me—scars and all. After all, Jesus had scars. His scars symbolize freedom, victory, strength, and His reckless love for us. I can reframe the way I look at my scars and accept them as good, and you can too!

Can you accept that perfection is unattainable and that it can become self-destructive? Are you aware that we can even become addicted to believing that we must look perfect? Many people struggle with self-image disorders and deal with addiction to plastic surgery. They even end up unrecognizable and sometimes mis-shapen from countless surgeries in an attempt to achieve perfection, yet they are never satisfied. Society tells us to have it all together, be perfect, and not let anyone see our weaknesses. Maybe for you, perfectionism was expected by a parent, caretaker, teacher, coach, or spouse, and that has made you a compulsive striver for perfection in your life. Striving is not success; it's self-defeating, unrealistic, and exhausting. Reframing your need to be perfect as progress over perfection is true success. It's time to let go of who you think you are supposed to be or who someone told you to be and embrace who you are—scars, mistakes, bad choices, and all.

How do we do that? We develop shame resilience that makes us more self-aware and willing to accept our scars as beautiful.

Developing Shame Resilience

Are you still "shoulding" all over yourself? Shaming yourself for being human and making mistakes? What if you were able to see yourself clearly without the shame? Debbie Ford, author of *The Dark Side of the Light Chasers* and *Why Good People Do Bad Things*, wrote, "Self-awareness is the ability to take an honest look at your life without any attachment to it being right or wrong, good or bad."[3]

Shame is intended to inform us that our positive feelings have been interrupted and we need to do something about it. Shame is a weapon used by the devil to corrupt and put distance in our relationship with God. The devil uses fear to silence us and shame to sabotage us. Because of this, we need to be reminded that shame was intended to be a signal to make us aware of our inadequacy and our need for a Savior in Jesus Christ. This is the essence of grace: Jesus took on our shame when He died on the cross. He not only endured shame, allowing Him to identify with ours, but He paid the price for our healing of sickness and disease and mental suffering. Hebrews 12:2 says He despised shame and conquered the humiliation of the cross. Jesus demonstrated His extravagant love for us through His suffering while showing us that shame does not have to have a hold on us. We can defeat shame because of His example and focus on the joy that is to come on the other side of working for freedom from shame. Take in this verse:

> We look away from the natural realm and we focus our attention and expectation onto Jesus who birthed faith within us and who leads us forward into faith's perfection. His example is this: Because his heart was focused on the joy of knowing that you would be his, he endured the agony of the cross and conquered its humiliation, and now sits exalted at the right hand of the throne of God! (Hebrews 12:2 TPT)

We have an opportunity to reframe the shame we have experienced in our lives and make it work for us rather than against us. By seeing our shame from another perspective, we can redeem our stories and what the enemy meant to harm us and take us out. It might seem counterintuitive, but vulnerability is the key to developing shame resistance.

Brené Brown wrote in her book *The Gifts of Imperfection: Let Go of Who You Think You're Supposed to Be and Embrace Who You Are*, "Owning our story can be hard but not nearly as difficult as spending our lives running from it. Embracing our vulnerabilities is risky but not nearly as dangerous as giving up on love and belonging and joy—the experiences that make us the most vulnerable. Only when we are brave enough to explore the darkness will we discover the infinite power of our light."[4]

What is in your story that you need to get vulnerable about with someone? What shame in your story needs to be uncovered so it can be reframed and redeemed and become a light for others? What shame are you hiding or denying that is holding you back from being the best and truest version of yourself? Shame can be experienced in many scenarios in our lives, all of which make us feel trapped or powerless in one way or another. Some experience shame about not being able to have children, of being single, of being unemployed, of having a home foreclosed on, of having a car repossessed, or of filing for bankruptcy. Are you hiding the abortions you've had, the number of sexual partners from the past, or even an STD you contracted as a result? What you reveal, you can heal.

Remember, shame loves secrecy and grows in hiding. Stop playing hide-and-seek with your shame. Stop hiding behind the fig leaves like Adam and Eve did. Look intentionally at the shame in your life with God's help. See where and what it is hiding that you need to be free from. There is freedom on the other side of dealing with our shame. Are you willing to work for it?

Brené Brown has outlined four key elements shared by people who are resilient to shame:

1. The ability to recognize and understand their shame triggers
2. High levels of critical awareness about their shame web
3. The willingness to reach out to others
4. The ability to speak shame[5]

As the Integrative Life Center wrote, "Shame is the fear of disconnection. Connection is why we as humans are here. Through connection with others, we develop purpose and meaning in our lives. For connection to happen, we must be seen by others. This is the concept of vulnerability."[6]

Isn't it crazy that we fear disconnection, yet it is fear that drives us from connecting with others? We fear connection because we don't want to get hurt, so as a result, we avoid it altogether. We don't want to feel rejected because of the painful memory of the parent who wasn't there for us or the spouse who abandoned us or cheated on us. We've been betrayed by people who were supposed to protect us and promised to love us till death do us part. We are paralyzed by fear to connect, yet it is the thing we long for the most.

Vulnerability requires us to take a leap of faith and risk being hurt. Isn't it better to love and have lost than never to have loved at all? To be vulnerable we need to allow ourselves to be seen as we truly are, warts, scars, imperfections, and all! To be vulnerable we must step out of our comfort zone into the unknown and accept the risk of being hurt. I get that this is hard. But this is also being brave. Vulnerability is strength and courage in action. Vulnerable people experience authentic connection with others because they are free to be who they are. They fight past fear in order to experience the authentic connection and belonging that we all desire deep down in the core of our humanity. The work to be vulnerable is worth it.

She Made Me

Have you ever looked at a picture of yourself as a child and had it bring something up for you that you feel shame about? Perhaps it reminded you of who you once were before awful things happened to you. You were reminded of the precious innocence of a child. Maybe as you looked at yourself, you thought, *Where did this child's innocence go?* Can you recall now the pain you were feeling in that moment?

I have thought the same things as I stared into the eyes of the little girl in the few baby pictures I have of myself. Those thoughts have come up for me as I looked at photos of the scantily clad young woman I was in high school. *She* was insecure and had no self-esteem. Having little fabric on her body gave her the attention she felt she needed from men because she didn't know her worth or how to esteem herself. The eyes of the woman in the photos were practically shut from all the alcohol *she* had consumed. Yup, that was me. So was the woman in the photos who couldn't even look at the camera because of the debilitating shame *she* walked in. The woman in all those pictures from childhood to adulthood, with all her issues, with all her shame, with all her pain—that woman was *me*!

The Irene I have seen in the mirror every day since day 38 in rehab is a *new creation*. The new Irene is free and can look back on the past Irene without regretting who she is. When I reframed the way I saw my past, I began to change my posture and self-esteem. I began to square my shoulders in confidence and walk in assurance that I am a child of God, forgiven, worthy, enough, and loved. That beautiful young girl made me who I am. *She* is who made *me*.

Acceptance of my story and the consequences of my choices, as well as the pain I caused, the drunken fights, and lying about alcohol, are all part of my miracle story. A disease that should have taken me out and kills so many people was not the end of me, but the beginning. Every photo I look at reminds me of the journey from *she* to *me*.

Healing the Child Within

Becoming the new Irene meant going back, with the help of counselors, to heal the little girl who experienced difficulty, hardship, trauma, and pain. I may have been developmentally stunted well into my thirties because of those experiences; however, now I walk in freedom as a functional adult because of taking time to heal and nurture the little girl in those photos. With my therapist in rehab, at home with my counselor, or in speaking with safe friends, I would revisit childhood memories. If I was sharing a memory with a friend and it brought up something that brought me discomfort, I would write it down to speak to my therapist about because it deserved deeper digging and work around it. You deserve healing from the pain you experienced in your childhood too.

I remember working with my counselor in the exercise of reparenting nine-year-old Irene regarding my issue with feeling abandoned by my father when he went overseas to work. I visualized her and put her on my lap. I hugged her and loved her by making her feel secure. I began to tell her that I understood how much it hurt to see her daddy leave, and why it felt like rejection and like he abandoned her. I said to her, with my counselor, "I understand that you miss him terribly and how painful this is." And I pictured myself wiping the tears from my nine-year-old self. I told her that her daddy loved her very much and wanted to take care of her. That he worked to make sure she had food to eat, clothes to wear, and a house to live in. I reassured her of his love and explained that he had to go to work in Africa because that is how he provided for his family. Through acknowledgment, empathy, and affirmation, little Irene began to heal and accept her new truth. Reparenting helped me heal repressed emotions I experienced growing up. It helped me identify the root causes of my abandonment and rejection issues and patterns in my adulthood.

This skill that I learned in counseling I can now apply on my own at home and in my everyday life. Such methods feel foreign to us because in our culture we don't usually take time to reflect, to see ourselves as children, to sit with our pain. But this is what heals us and reminds us that we can accept ourselves and be whole.

Now when I revisit memories of heartbreak, I acknowledge the emotions. I listen to the thoughts and experiences of the little girl and empathize with her. I don't leave her there in her mess, though!

> Reparenting helped me heal repressed emotions I experienced growing up. It helped me identify the root causes of my abandonment and rejection issues and patterns in my adulthood.

I help her experience truth. I reach out to a counselor as needed, and I journal any dreams that I feel may reveal something I need to revisit in therapy. I have even written letters as a therapeutic way to heal my inner child. You will be amazed at how much self-awareness, healing, and self-compassion you will develop doing this type of work.

In year three of my sobriety, I was aware that I was beginning to exhibit symptoms of being a dry drunk. I was going to fewer meetings, wasn't in counseling as much, and felt depressed and anxious. The pity parties of not being able to drink ever again were sending me to a place of grief. I was angry and sad and jealous of normal drinkers. I started having dreams about drinking that felt so real I could taste the chardonnay. I knew I was in trouble because of what I had learned from the old-timer in AA, and I prayed for God to speak to me and help me. But I didn't stop with prayer—I also got my butt back in meetings regularly. I don't believe it was by chance that I happened upon a book by Annie Grace called *This*

Naked Mind: Control Alcohol, Find Freedom, Discover Happiness & Change Your Life.[7] God set me up to read this book, and at just the right moment something jumped off the page at me and practically slapped me in the face. This is when my "have to stop drinking" became my "I get to not drink."

In one moment, everything changed, and I woke up! I was conscious again. *I get to* not wake up in shame and remorse with a nauseating hangover. *I get to* be present to enjoy people without needing the crutch of the false liquid confidence of alcohol. I was able to reframe the way I viewed not drinking. *I get to* not wake up hungover anymore, not remembering what I did or said the night before. *I get to* enjoy the power of no remorse, shame, or regret from binge drinking. *I get to* not make a fool of myself by slurring my words and being loud and obnoxious. *I get to* not fear killing or hurting myself—or, worse, others—behind the wheel of a car while driving drunk. *I get to* not fear consequences like jail time. *I get to* wake up happy and grateful, ready to begin each day rather than dread it. *I get to* live in forgiveness and acceptance by God and my loved ones. *I get to* not drink. *I get to* remember enjoyable moments and not struggle to forget the bad ones. *I get to be free!*

The "get tos" of life are what help us reframe shame. We *get to* be present in our emotions and deal with them and be present for ourselves and heal in recovery. I can look in the mirror and believe, *I get to be me.* And I finally like me.

No Longer Anonymous

Here's another way to put it: You're here to be light, bringing out the God-colors in the world. God is not a secret to be kept.

We're going public with this, as public as a city on a hill. If I make you light-bearers, you don't think I'm going to hide you under a bucket, do you? I'm putting you on a light stand. Now that I've put you there on a hilltop, on a light stand—shine! Keep open house; be generous with your lives. By opening up to others, you'll prompt people to open up with God, this generous Father in heaven. (Matthew 5:14–16 MSG)

There comes a time when we are ready to share our stories and our journey. This looks different for each of us, and that's okay. With the help of our support team, we can determine when we feel ready to open up our lives to others. Sunday, March 4, 2018, was the day I finally felt I had a peace to go public and share my story with our church. My brilliant husband asked me to speak in a sermon series he titled "This Is My Story." He asked various people to share on Sunday mornings about how they had overcome obstacles in their lives, and my particular Sunday was a defining moment in time when I would be vulnerable and transparent with my church family in hopes of inspiring others to overcome shame in their issues. My story was out! The grip of shame loosened on me as I shared my story and no longer had anything to hide.

Jimmy always believed in me more than I believed in myself and seemed to find ways to make me shine. He believed the scripture as it says that we must go public and be salt and light to the earth. Our lives were about helping others, and we could do that with our story of recovering as a family. We felt strongly about sharing with the world how God had redeemed our relationship and rescued us from our dysfunction.

This particular Sunday we would not just talk about it, but we would be about it. As we went public with the pain and shame of our story of redemption as a family, we believed it would prompt others to open up with God, our generous Father in heaven, who was there to meet them, heal them, restore them, and lead them on a path of healing and recovery.

With my family and friends sitting guard front and center at church, and me nervously sweating profusely, I confessed to the congregation, "My name is Irene, and I am a grateful recovering alcoholic. I am two years and three months sober." The entire congregation stood to their feet and cheered, and people all over the room were crying. When they sat down, I began to lay out my journey into addiction and the way out of it. The energy I felt and the confidence exuding from me was unparalleled by anything I had experienced before, and I knew God was shining through me. *What?* I thought, *Could this really be happening?* I wasn't expecting people to cheer! In my mind, I had catastrophized the worst scenarios that everyone would reject me. Instead, I received empathy. People identified with my story and appreciated my vulnerability, and some desperately wanted freedom for themselves. Many admitted they needed help and got sober that day. Many identified their brokenness and started the road to recovery. Just as the stories in the small circle in rehab had given me permission to be honest, I sensed that my sharing gave people permission to admit their issues as well. Our community was inspired by my family's story of redemption to pursue their own healing. It didn't destroy our church when people found out. In fact, our church grew steadily over time as we became more transparent about God's redemptive power changing our lives.

I began to receive countless testimonies and messages from people saying that because of our vulnerability as leaders, they felt they could come to our church and receive God's grace for themselves as well. Through my openly sharing my weaknesses, I brought glory to God for what He did in my life and became a portal for God's power to work in others! Wow! My shame was being transformed into purpose. Now I understand that my weaknesses don't define me, and I am not defeated by them. Rather, I can delight in them and celebrate them because they are a testimony of God's power at work in me. I love how 2 Corinthians 12:9–10 expresses this in The Passion Translation: "My grace is always more than enough for you, and my power finds its full expression through your weakness."

So I will celebrate my weaknesses, for when I'm weak I sense more deeply the mighty power of Christ living in me. So I'm *not defeated* by my weakness, but delighted! For when I feel my weakness and endure mistreatment—when I'm surrounded with troubles on every side and face persecution *because of my love* for Christ—I am made yet stronger. For my weakness becomes a portal to God's power.

If you believe this, your shame can be reframed.

Finding and Accepting God's Grace

I believed unconsciously for a long time, even as I went to church and served God vocationally, that His grace applied to others but somehow I was too far gone. His grace didn't apply to me. My addiction to alcohol and distorted internal belief and value system only magnified this untrue belief. I felt that I was not worthy enough to receive this grace that God offers.

Grace is unmerited favor, which means that we don't deserve it and there is nothing we can do to earn it. It is freely given to us. It is ours because God so loved us that He gave His one and only Son that we may be forgiven of our sins and have eternal life (John 3:16).

Grace is difficult to accept even for the most professional and seasoned Christians because we have difficulty wrapping our minds around the notion of such unconditional love and acceptance. What a massive love God has that He would give up His only Son to die a horrific, humiliating, and painful death so we could be forgiven of our sin nature as human beings. The hymn "Amazing Grace" is sung in churches around the world. It speaks to how the amazing grace of God can relieve our hearts from fear. Fear of what? Fear of disconnection from God. Fear that we are not enough, which is the essence of shame.

Having questions and doubts is a perfectly normal part of our spiritual journey and discovery. Jesus treated people who had doubts with compassion and valued their questions, as described in countless ways throughout the Bible. He didn't hesitate to show His own humanity by sharing His emotion of sadness as He wept when Lazarus died. Jesus asked God to take the circumstances of His crucifixion away because He feared the pain of what was to come in His suffering on the cross. Yet after He prayed, cried, and sought God, He surrendered His will to the will of God, which meant dying for the sins of mankind. Jesus cried out to God before He was crucified. He experienced peace and the grace necessary to carry out His assignment. That grace saved mankind by ensuring our everlasting connection with God. Jesus values and can handle our questions and doubts. He has compassion for us as we process them.

When we surrender to God's grace, as Jesus did, deciding to turn our will over to Him and His care, we can accept all the grace and forgiveness He has to offer. Why do we resist submitting to the authority of a God who loves us? Just like Adam and Eve in the garden, fear and shame hinder our capacity to trust God, to believe that His ways are better for us. Thankfully, God is love, and in His love, God gave humans the power of choice. We have free will. We get to choose to believe in God or not. We get to choose to surrender to *our* will and desires (which much of the time doesn't work out so well for us), *or* we can decide to choose to surrender to the safety found in God's will and plan for us that is always good (Jeremiah 29:11; Romans 12:2).

Are you ready to accept God's grace and forgiveness once and for all?

Why Jesus?

Do you have questions about salvation and faith in Jesus? Are you wondering what you need to be "saved from" when you hear people use the term *saved* to describe their salvation experience? Are you wondering *how* you can have a personal relationship with Jesus and press the Reset button on your life and receive salvation? Take a moment now and turn to the appendix for a special prayer written for you to receive Jesus Christ as your Savior, Redeemer, and forgiver of your sins. He promises new life to us, that we can become born again, new creations in Christ.

Ownership of our flaws brings us to our knees, keeping us humble and aware of our brokenness and need for a savior. When Jesus Christ redeems us and forgives us through the work of the cross, we are free to be our authentic selves, flaws and all, knowing that we don't have to do this life alone. God is with us, guiding us and giving us grace and strength to overcome our weaknesses every moment of every day.

A Daily Battle

Recovery from shame is a daily battle. And over time the battle gets easier. Shame doesn't have to defeat us or harm us. We can become shame resilient if we work toward vulnerability. Remember, vulnerability is the remedy for shame. As Brené Brown said, "Vulnerability is the birthplace of love, belonging, joy, courage, empathy, and creativity. It is the source of hope, empathy, accountability, and authenticity."[8]

My prayer and hope for you is that this concept of progress over perfection frees you to be imperfect! I pray it fuels you to accept your imperfections and be gentler with yourself as well as have more grace for other imperfect people. Be compassionate with yourself. You are not a failure because you made a mistake. Remind yourself that mistakes are opportunities to grow and learn so we don't repeat them. It's time to accept that our mistakes are sometimes a necessary detour (not a dead end) to our purpose being fulfilled. There is nothing more freeing than not having anything to hide.

Recovery Is for Everyone

We now know that recovery applies to everyone because we all have struggles, dysfunction in our upbringing, and stress that will continue to happen in our lives daily. Trauma is real, but so is resilience.

You are stronger and more resilient than you think! It is up to us to make the choice to handle life in a way that benefits us. We can learn to manage the stress, grief, change, life transitions, and situations that come our way both past and present and become flexible to pivot as changes come our way. We can learn to treat the real source of our issues and find solutions to any problem that comes our way. We can choose to forgive and accept that reconciliation will be a process. We don't need to wait to be forgiven by others to forgive ourselves. Forgiveness is a choice; reconciliation is a process. It may not look the way we thought it would, but reconciliation is ours for the taking.

I meet people all over the country when I travel, and many send me messages on social media saying they have a desire to stop drinking or using a particular substance, person, or thing to satiate or medicate themselves. However, after acknowledging that they have a problem, asking for help, and receiving my recommendations, many offer excuses as to why they can't do what it takes to get sober. I can hear the codependency loud and clear as they say some true things, such as that finances are an issue and they can't get to rehab or that they can't leave their kids for that long. I know, I said the same things. Problem is, my kids were already losing me the longer I prolonged getting the help I needed. I was killing myself slowly. By making the financial sacrifice and getting help, I gave them the best gift ever—a healthy mom. Making excuses about why not to get help is more about shame and the manipulative nature of addiction to keep you sick.

More free resources than you may realize are available to you or your loved one, but you have to research which program best suits your needs or the needs of your loved one's recovery journey. Remember, recovery applies to everyone and will look different for us all. It will be messy, exhausting, and downright hard sometimes. Here is the deal: you can make your own misery, or you can make yourself strong. The amount of work is the same. You can choose to stop making excuses and do something today to change your life even if it is as small as choosing to get into counseling or to stop eating fried food or sweets. Getting vulnerable with another person is hard, and abstaining from food we love is hard. I get it. But staying isolated and left to your own stinking thinking is making you depressed. You feel shame and pain when you have to get two seats on an airplane because you are overweight. Both are hard. The suffering is the same. How badly do you want to get well? Choose your "hard" today.

For those who have a loved one still in an addiction, I hope you realize how important your own recovery and need to establish boundaries is. You can't do it alone, and help is available for you also. You are worth the care and investment in your healing. Dealing with the impact of the addiction on you will help set you free, and you, too, can get unstuck and thrive in your own life even if your loved one doesn't get sober. You are worth the investment of discovering ways to process your hurts, hang-ups, and habits to keep your emotional health in order. Remember, the loved ones of those in addiction are just as sick emotionally as the person in the addiction. Don't forget about *you* in it all.

Those of you who are leaders in the church may still be wondering, *Will this discredit me in my ministry if people find out I was struggling while leading or that I still am struggling?* I thought about that, too, and tortured myself over it. Bottom line is, I got help. I got honest. I got well, and now I help others do the same. If I keep worrying about what others will think, I will stay in the bondage that led me to drink in the first place—the disease of codependency.

It's time to admit it. You cannot quit it *until* you admit it! God's power can't come in to make you strong until you admit you are weak! Don't allow fear and shame to hold you back from all that God desires for you and those in your sphere of influence to experience through your healing and redemption story. Choose progress over perfection any day!

Become the Safe Person You Need

In the recovery journey, we sometimes have to walk away from the people and places that enable our behavior or hinder our decisions to change. It's time to own our responsibility to grow and make decisions that further that growth. Not everyone will grow and change with you. Not everyone will like the boundaries you set or the choices you make to recover. But you can honor your convictions to change. You can become a safe person in the process.

A safe person is someone who admits their flaws and apologizes for mistakes. They are transparent, dependable, and honest. Safe people are accountable in their own recovery journey, and if you're looking for someone to trust, look for a person with the credibility of several years of sobriety under their belt. Look for someone who is life giving when providing feedback, who doesn't tear you down or shame you. A safe person won't hesitate to have hard conversations with you to hold you accountable if you have allowed them into the vulnerable places of your life. They demonstrate consistency in understanding boundaries, because they consistently show you that they respect and honor yours and will not allow you to wreck theirs. There is safety in having accountability.

Unsafe people do the opposite of these things. They use your secrets and vulnerable moments they've witnessed to hurt you. Other characteristics include name-calling, gaslighting, blaming you for being abused, or frequently dismissing your emotions. This happens a lot in the dysfunctional romantic relationship cycle and in situations where someone holds power or authority over us. Unsafe people who have hurt us make us wonder about ourselves, *Is it me? What is wrong with me, and what am I doing wrong? Why do people keep leaving me, hurting me, using me, betraying me?*

According to Brené Brown's research, "Trust—an integral component of all thriving relationships and workplaces—can be broken up into seven key elements; boundaries, reliability, accountability, vault (confidentiality), integrity, non-judgment and generosity."[9] Become the person of integrity and trust you need in your life, for someone else.

The promises of AA still ring true for me as I work my program of recovery with all my heart and soul. The promises of recovery happen sometimes quickly and sometimes slowly, depending on each individual and how we apply ourselves to working the steps of our recovery journey. I pray that God will give you a vision of the healed version of yourself. A picture of what life could be like as you confront the things that have been holding you back from experiencing the freedom you deserve.

I encourage you to write down your journey so you can come back to it over time and see how much progress you are making as you evolve and do the work. As you gain courage to share your story and experiences, you will not only inspire others but quite possibly save lives as well. So many people are suffering, thinking they are alone in their struggles, and it doesn't have to be that way. We all have a unique story and something to offer others. There's a reason every recovery meeting opens with someone's story. As we share, we help others and lose interest in selfish things. Serving others helps to keep us sober. Our greatest misery can become our greatest ministry! It is never about us. When we overcome, we help others overcome. Maya Angelou said, "When you get, give. When you learn, teach."[10] It's never about us! It's about serving others. Addiction makes us selfish, and by serving others we reverse that programming. Make it practical—encourage someone else through a kind gesture or comforting words today. Send a text to someone to check on them. "Let us think of ways to motivate one another to acts of love and good works" (Hebrews 10:24 NLT).

Finding ways to serve others while we are recovering is so important. Take part in service opportunities at your recovery meeting, volunteer in your community, or partner with a local church that does outreach in the community. Use what God gave you—your natural gifts and talents. Don't overthink it; just find somewhere you can serve and be a blessing to someone else. Healed people heal other people. Our purpose once we receive God's grace, healing, and forgiveness is to go share those things with all those suffering and longing to receive that peace and healing we have. We gotta give it away!

The apostle Paul wrote in Galatians 6:4–5, "Make a careful exploration of who you are and the work you have been given, and then sink yourself into that. Don't be impressed with yourself. Don't compare yourself with others. Each of you must take responsibility for doing the creative best you can with your own life" (MSG).

God Has a Great Purpose for Your Life!

Jeremiah 29:11–13 says, "'For I know the plans I have for you,' declares the LORD, 'plans to prosper you and not to harm you, plans to give you hope and a future. Then you will call on me and come and pray to me, and I will listen to you. You will seek me and find me when you seek me with all your heart.'"

What's even more powerful about this Scripture is that when the Lord declared it through the prophet Jeremiah, the people were not in a good place. They were hurting, broken, enslaved, and figuring out how to live again in a land that was unfamiliar and scary. The shame of their grief and loss, hurt and harm could have overshadowed the good work God wanted to do in them and through them. This is true in recovery as well. Whatever depths of despair you are in, no matter how messy your recovery is, God still has a purpose and a plan to use all you have been through for a greater purpose.

In my final words, I want to remind you that you can do this. God is with you, and He is for you. I am rooting for you. You are not alone. You can't heal a lifetime of pain overnight. Be gentle with yourself; rebuilding yourself takes time. It's okay to be scared; that means you are about to do something really brave!

Trust the process. Do this for you, not for anyone else. Honor yourself. Love yourself. You deserve it. Survival mode helped you survive, but you weren't meant to live there. It's a new day with new promises and goodness to experience.

Get the help you need to be whole. One of the greatest mental freedoms is not caring what anyone else thinks of you. As you journey, let go of what you thought should happen and live in what is happening. Be present. Stay in the moment—the future is overwhelming, and besides, you don't have to live there because the future hasn't happened yet. Lay down your worry and your hurry. You get to decide what today will look like for yourself. That is enough to deal with.

Remember that healed people heal people. Get honest, get real, be vulnerable, ask for help, get help, do the work, get healthy, then go out into the world and give away what you have learned and received. Give it away! Reframe your shame and do the work to get free so you can help set others free!

Letters to Readers

To: Christian Leaders

It's Okay Not to Be Okay

Our congregations and churches are full of people suffering with mental health problems and addiction. Why are we not talking more about this in the church? Pastors and leaders struggle too! After all, we are human. Like me, some pastors and leaders, and their congregations, deal with addictions openly. Many more are pretending they don't exist! It is only a matter of time before the truth eventually comes out and leaves them, their families, and communities to face the consequences of their undealt-with struggles, whether it is mental health, trauma, addiction, or something else. These struggles, whether they are hidden or in public view, are still a real and dangerous threat to our communities and families.

Many leaders, who may have already been close to their tipping point prior to the COVID-19 pandemic, have found themselves completely overwhelmed. They are living outside of their normal ability to tolerate stress, leading many to destructive behaviors and even suicide as they grapple desperately for ways to cope. When we deny the brokenness of our own humanity and partner that with the dangerous lie that we are somehow supposed to be immune from struggles, dysfunction, hardship, and addictions because we are in the public eye, we are prideful and headed toward danger. Just because we are leaders and people look up to us, we believe the lie that moral failure means the end for us. As if the Bible is not filled with people who made terrible choices and discovered a saving, redeeming, delivering God! People still need heroes in their lives who are not trying to be saviors but are able to set an example of how to walk in integrity. There's a great need for people whom others can look up to, who don't collapse due to the effects and/or consequences of their hidden issues. You can create a culture that no perfect people are allowed in your church or organization, where you embrace your humanity rather than shaming people for being human. We can teach our congregations that our failures don't define us; rather, we are defined by what we do when we rise after we fall, and we can't do this without the grace and mercy of God.

We must get well so we can lead others well. Through recovery, therapy, and reciprocal relationships, we can offload the junk that has been weighing us down so we can show others how to get real and get free through the power of Jesus Christ. Jesus went hard on religious leaders who pretended to be perfect and demanded that others do the same. In Matthew 23:4 He said, "They crush people with unbearable religious demands and never lift a finger to ease the burden" (NLT) and in verse 25 He added, "What sorrow awaits you teachers of religious law and you Pharisees. Hypocrites! For you are so careful to clean the outside of the cup and the dish, but inside you are filthy—full of greed and self-indulgence!" (NLT).

Perfection is a crushing demand, not just for you, but for the people in your life. It is not the way of Jesus, who invites all who are weary to come to Him and He will give us rest, because His yoke is easy and His burden is light (Matthew 11:28, 30). Who told you that you had to keep up the appearance of having it all together, being perfect, that you aren't supposed to have struggles? Matthew 23:25 warns of the misery we will bring upon ourselves when we are so careful to keep up the facade that everything is shiny, clean, perfect, and looking good in our lives while the truth is we are dying on the inside. Can you remember who you were before the world told you who you "should" be?

Pastors and clergy leaders, it really is okay not to be okay! People in our congregations, especially in the younger generations coming up behind us, long for transparency and vulnerability. Unattainable perfection is no longer an acceptable aspiration for young people. I don't know about you, but I am so over it! It is exhausting to rely more on myself than on the God I serve. This passage from 2 Corinthians speaks to me, because Paul, a man delivered from pride and self-righteousness, wrote honestly and hopefully about learning to rely on God:

> In fact, we expected to die. But as a result, we stopped relying on ourselves and learned to rely only on God, who raises the dead. And he did rescue us from mortal danger, and he will rescue us again. We have placed our confidence in him, and he will continue to rescue us. And you are helping us by praying for us. Then many people will give thanks because God has graciously answered so many prayers for our safety. (2 Corinthians 1:9–11 NLT)

What if we began to take responsibility for our character flaws and to own our brokenness and resist shame over our need for recovery? I believe this is a path toward freedom.

As a senior pastor in my church for ten years, I know the weight you carry. You are not alone. Don't do life and ministry alone. I implore you to seek emotional healing and pursue God to heal your own brokenness. The gifts and calling of God are irrevocable (Romans 11:29). You will not be disqualified by admitting your weaknesses. As you seek wholeness and healing, you will not only get free but partner with God to set others free! Keep fighting the good fight of faith. Do the work and trust the process.

To: Families of Those Struggling with Addiction

You Don't Deserve This

First of all, I want to acknowledge the pain and suffering you are going through with your loved one dealing with an addiction. I am truly sorry for all parties involved, but I am especially sorry for how their addiction has impacted you. I am sorry for the nights you have stayed up late anxiously waiting for your loved one to return home safely. I am sorry you have had to see them inebriated and blacking out and have stood helpless while emergency services worked to revive your loved one from an overdose, suicide attempt, alcohol poisoning, or something else.

You don't deserve to be stolen from, lied to, or manipulated.

You don't deserve to be called profane words or violated physically by your loved one under the influence.

Cleaning up the collateral damage created by your loved one

is not your life sentence. You may never get the acknowledgment from the person who has hurt you, but I want you to know that you can move forward and heal even if you never get the apology you deserve. You are not crazy for loving them past their behaviors, because you likely remember who they were before their brains were hijacked by addiction.

Don't give up on praying for your loved one and encouraging them to get help. While it remains important that they get help, you can't control whether they choose to or not. I encourage you to make yourself and your healing the number one priority. Family members can be just as sick emotionally as the person in the addiction.

Lean into your own healing and emotional well-being. It's okay to say no, communicate ultimatums, and assert boundaries to protect yourself. You are not betraying your loved one by saying no when boundaries are being violated. Their trust can be earned back as they get sober and demonstrate they are willing to do the work to get free.

Celebrate every win, every meeting they attend to stay sober and get healthy. True change comes with time and repetition, and your encouragement is key to helping them get free from the shame of recovery. Remember, even if your loved one relapses and/ or doesn't get sober, it doesn't mean you have to take or allow it in your space, heart, or home. You can move forward and take care of yourself emotionally. You deserve it!

Acknowledgments

*G*od, thank You for being a good Father to me. Thank You for sending Your Son, Jesus, that I might have eternal life with You and be rescued from myself. Thank You for Your grace, mercy, and redemptive power that has set me free. Thank You for anointing me, calling me, healing me, and giving me life. Thank You for a second chance at life and for propelling me into my purpose through using every hard season of my life for my good and the good of others. Thank You for never leaving me even in my darkest times and showing me there is always a way forward. I promise to give away all the love and knowledge You have given me so I can help set others free. I pray that through my testimony, they may know You and see the beauty of Your endless, reckless, and extravagant love for us all.

Jimmy, you are truly the love of my life. I do not believe there are enough words in the English vocabulary to describe my intense love and gratitude for you. I would not be who I am today without you by my side, always believing the best in me when it wasn't easy and I wasn't able to see any goodness in myself. You have pushed and fought through the hardest situations life has thrown our way. You are a finisher! You have done the work and overcome your own struggles, and I am so proud of you! I am eternally grateful for your massive, generous heart and your love for God, me, and our family. Thank you for loving me past my yuck and being my homie, lover, and best friend. Now and forever, at the end of the day, it's just me and you! We are two equally crazy people who are equally committed, and now we have been made one. Two = One! I love you for life!

Kayla, Jaden, and Maya, thank you for making me a mommy! I will forever cherish having the opportunity to be your mother. Thank you for forgiving me, loving me, and encouraging my sobriety by enthusiastically and genuinely cheering me on in my journey of recovery. Your ability to be honest in sharing your hearts with me has inspired me to do the same. I believe in you guys. Each of you is a brave soul. I love each of you and the unique things that make you individually awesome! Thank you for journeying with me and embracing your individual story as well as our family story. I see you helping many through sharing what we have been through. You are world changers! Rollins Five forever!

Dr. Carol Robbins, you are a godsend as a therapist! Thank you for confronting us and challenging our dysfunction individually and as a family. You were the first person to help me see how bad off I was in my addiction and shame and to give me the hard push I needed to get help and finally go to rehab and deal with my alcoholism. This saved my life! Through Imago Relationship Therapy, you helped Jimmy and me stop the destructive dance of bad communication in our marriage. Thank you for giving us the tools we needed to be a part of healing each other and taking our marriage to a level of intimacy we never thought possible. We are so grateful as a family for your help in understanding ADD and

ADHD and how it impacted our relationships, and for giving us the tools we needed to live our best lives emotionally. You helped us embrace and deal with our mental health as a family, and for that we are forever changed for the better and forever grateful.

Mommy and Daddy, thank you for giving me life, and for all the experiences that have shaped me for the good, the bad, and the ugly. They are all valued and are a part of who I am today. I will never forget or take for granted the sacrifices you made for me and our family to give us all we had. Till we meet again in heaven, I love you.

To my siblings, Yvonne, Karen, Paul, Denis, and Brian—I want to thank you for loving me with a fierceness even when you didn't understand me and I was hard to love. Thank you for loving me just the way I am. You all mean the world to me! I also appreciate all the incredible nieces and nephews, sisters-in-law and brothers-in-law relationships that have blessed our family beyond measure.

To my father-in-law and mother-in-law, James and Varle Rollins, I am forever grateful for your love and acceptance of me as a daughter and your endless support and prayers for our family. Thank you for being the best in-laws a girl could ask for. Tonya, my SIL, you are the best! I love you and your beautiful mini-me's.

To my church family (i5 City), thank you for living beyond yourself, loving beyond your preferences, and laughing beyond your struggles. I will never forget you.

My pastors, Dino and DeLynn Rizzo, I thank God He sent you to Jimmy and me when we needed you most! Thank you for standing by us and never giving up on us. The countless phone calls, encouragement, and support will never be forgotten. We love and appreciate your relationship. We are family!

Elders Noland and Terry Henson, you have consistently been

my biggest cheerleaders. I value your prayers, encouragement, and support more than I can ever express. Thank you for believing in Jimmy and me and pushing us to be who God called us to be.

To my friends—you know who you are. I don't need to list your names. You will know you are part of this acknowledgment and thank-you because you loved me and my family through our toughest season. You brought meals, prayed for and encouraged us, and told us to keep pressing on and never give up. You cared for my family while I was gone to rehab. Thank you for saying the hard things and holding me accountable for hurting you when I hid my drinking from you. Thank you for sharing your stories with me. They inspired me to get open about mine. You all have been such a gift and inspiration to me, and I love that we are on this life journey together. Through the hard conversations, listening to me process, holding me accountable, and praying for me, our friendships have grown, and I am better because of you all. Thank you for sticking by my side in the darkest valleys and on the mountaintops. I love you all!

Ladies of my OPAAT AA home group, I am grateful for your demonstration of courage in fighting for sobriety, working the steps of the program, and reaching out to others to help them on their journey. Your stories have inspired me and taught me so much. I am forever grateful for your part in my journey of recovery.

Celebrate Recovery small group—*we do the work!* You all make me better! I am challenged and accountable, and I continue to grow as we do the work together. Such vulnerable and sacred space we have together, and I honor you all for richly impacting my life.

Andi Andrew, you have served as a friend and a midwife in my life. You have helped me push forth my purpose, and I would never have written this book if it wasn't for your guidance, sharing of resources, encouragement, and prayers. I'm so honored to lead the She Is Free movement with you and lead others into freedom together!

Ashley Abercrombie, speaking of being a midwife, this book would not have happened without your encouragement and coaching. Thank you for believing in me!

The Meadows treatment center—for every doctor, nurse, psychologist, and teacher I had the privilege of meeting, thank you for being a part of my journey. Thank you for showing me the way to lead and live a better life. A sober life.

Friends at The Meadows, I will never forget how you loved me back to life. Thank you for your empathy toward me when I was in denial about my alcoholism. Thank you for explaining and sharing the nature of the insidious disease of alcoholism and your own experiences of strength and hope. You inspired me to get well! I am specifically grateful that you never shamed me, but lovingly accepted me while encouraging me to deal with the reality and consequences of my addiction.

APPENDIX A

Additional Resources

- A Place of HOPE counseling center
  http://www.aplaceofhope.com
- Al-Anon World Service
  http://www.al-alnon.org/
- Alcoholics Anonymous World Service (AA)
  http://www.aa.org
- Celebrate Recovery Official
  http://www.celebraterecovery.com
- Center on Addiction
  http://www.centeronaddiction.org
- Certified Sex Addiction Therapist
  http://www.iitap.com/
- Co-Dependents Anonymous World Service (CODA)
  http://www.coda.org
- CrossRoads Counseling of the Rockies
  http://www.crossroadscounseling.net

ADDITIONAL RESOURCES

- EMDR Practitioners
  http://www.emdr.com
- Emotional Healing and Therapy and Workshops
  https://onsiteworkshops.com/
- Honey Lake Clinic Christian Counseling Center
  http://www.honeylake.clinic
- Imago Relationship Therapists
  https://www.imagorelationshipswork.com
- Men's Sex Addiction Treatment Center
  http://www.gentlepathmeadows.com
- Narcotics Anonymous (NA)
  http://www.na.org
- Online Therapy Options
  www.betterhelp.com
- SMART Recovery
  http://www.smartrecovery.org
- Somatic Experiencing Practitioners
  http://traumahealing.com/somaticexperiencing/practitioner
  -directory.html
- Substance Abuse and Mental Health Services Administration
  http://www.samhsa.gov
- Suicide Hotline
  1-800-273-8255
  http://www.suicidepreventionlifeline.org
- The Meadows Treatment Center
  http://www.themeadows.com
- Therapist Options via Psychology Today
  http://www.psychologytoday.com/

APPENDIX B

Receiving Salvation

Salvation is a gift from God to man. Man can never make up for his sin by self-improvement or good works. Only by trusting in Jesus Christ as God's offer of forgiveness can man be saved from sin's penalty. Eternal life begins the moment one receives Jesus Christ into his life by faith.

If you say with your mouth that Jesus is Lord, and believe in your heart that God raised Him from the dead, you will be saved from the punishment of sin. When we believe in our hearts, we are made right with God. We tell with our mouth how we were saved from the punishment of sin. (Romans 10:9–10 NLV)

Salvation Prayer

Lord Jesus, I need Your help. I've tried everything I know to do, and I cannot help myself. I've realized I cannot save myself, no matter what I do. I am ready to turn my life over to a higher power, and I am ready to trust You as my Savior and Lord. Thank You that You love me just as I am. I surrender my way to You. I believe that You are the Son of God, who died on the cross for my sins. I believe in the resurrection, that You died and rose again. I believe that in receiving You as my Savior, You will fill me now with the Holy Spirit, who is my advocate and guide, my comfort and help. Thank You for giving me the confidence that You are always with me, that no matter my mistakes and failures, You will never leave me. Thank You for the gift of eternal life, and the hope for freedom that I find in You. I trust You, and I welcome You to move in my life. In Jesus' name, amen.

Congratulations! Salvation is the best decision you will ever make! God is ready to meet you where your faith is, no matter how small that may be, and no matter where you are in your spiritual journey. Just as we make effort in any relationship that is important to us, to nurture and grow it, so does our relationship with Jesus Christ. Finding a local church where you can be part of a community to grow in and develop your relationship with God, learning to read the Bible and understanding God, is a great next step! Here are some scriptures to help you on your journey.

APPENDIX C

Scriptures to Read

Psalm 51 (A Psalm of Repentance)

Have mercy on me, O God,
     according to your unfailing love;
according to your great compassion
     blot out my transgressions.
Wash away all my iniquity
     and cleanse me from my sin.

For I know my transgressions,
     and my sin is always before me.
Against you, you only, have I sinned
     and done what is evil in your sight;
so you are right in your verdict
     and justified when you judge.

Surely I was sinful at birth,
   sinful from the time my mother
   conceived me.
Yet you desired faithfulness even in the womb;
   you taught me wisdom in that secret
   place.

Cleanse me with hyssop, and I will be clean;
   wash me, and I will be whiter
   than snow.
Let me hear joy and gladness;
   let the bones you have crushed rejoice.
Hide your face from my sins
   and blot out all my iniquity.

Create in me a pure heart, O God,
   and renew a steadfast spirit
   within me.
Do not cast me from your presence
   or take your Holy Spirit from me.
Restore to me the joy of your salvation
   and grant me a willing spirit, to
   sustain me.

Then I will teach transgressors your ways,
   so that sinners will turn back to you.
Deliver me from the guilt of bloodshed, O God,
   you who are God my Savior,
   and my tongue will sing of your
   righteousness.

Open my lips, Lord,
>and my mouth will declare your
>praise.
You do not delight in sacrifice, or I would
>bring it; you do not take pleasure in burnt
>offerings.
My sacrifice, O God, is a broken spirit;
>a broken and contrite heart
>you, God, will not despise.

May it please you to prosper Zion,
>to build up the walls of Jerusalem.
Then you will delight in the sacrifices of the
>righteous,
>in burnt offerings offered whole;
>then bulls will be offered on your altar.

Psalm 139 (A Promise of God's Presence)

You have searched me, LORD,
and you know me.
You know when I sit and when I rise;
you perceive my thoughts from afar.
You discern my going out and my lying down;
you are familiar with all my ways.
Before a word is on my tongue
you, LORD, know it completely.
You hem me in behind and before,
and you lay your hand upon me.
Such knowledge is too wonderful for me,
too lofty for me to attain.

Where can I go from your Spirit?
Where can I flee from your presence?
If I go up to the heavens, you are there;
if I make my bed in the depths, you are
there.
If I rise on the wings of the dawn,
if I settle on the far side of the sea,
even there your hand will guide me,
your right hand will hold me fast.
If I say, "Surely the darkness will hide me
and the light become night around me,"
even the darkness will not be dark to you;
the night will shine like the day,
for darkness is as light to you.

For you created my inmost being;
>> you knit me together in my
>> mother's womb.
I praise you because I am fearfully and
>> wonderfully made;
>> your works are wonderful,
>> I know that full well.
My frame was not hidden from you
>> when I was made in the secret place,
>> when I was woven together in the
>> depths of the earth.
Your eyes saw my unformed body;
>> all the days ordained for me were
>> written in your book
>> before one of them came to be.
How precious to me are your thoughts, God!
>> How vast is the sum of them!
Were I to count them,
>> they would outnumber the grains
>> of sand—
>> when I awake, I am still with you.

If only you, God, would slay the wicked!
>> Away from me, you who are
>> bloodthirsty!
They speak of you with evil intent;
>> your adversaries misuse your name.
Do I not hate those who hate you, LORD,
>> and abhor those who are in rebellion
>> against you?

I have nothing but hatred for them;
I count them my enemies.
Search me, God, and know my heart;
test me and know my anxious
thoughts.
See if there is any offensive way in me,
and lead me in the way everlasting.

Additional Verses

Romans 10:9

If you declare with your mouth, "Jesus is Lord," and believe in your heart that God raised him from the dead, you will be saved.

John 14:6

Jesus answered, "I am the way and the truth and the life. No one comes to the Father except through me."

Ephesians 2:8–9

For it is by grace you have been saved, through faith—and this is not from yourselves, it is the gift of God—not by works, so that no one can boast.

Titus 3:5

He saved us, not because of righteous things we had done, but because of his mercy. He saved us through the washing of rebirth and renewal by the Holy Spirit.

Acts 16:30–33

He then brought them out and asked, "Sirs, what must I do to be saved?"

They replied, "Believe in the Lord Jesus, and you will be saved—you and your household." Then they spoke the word of the Lord to him and to all the others in his house. At that hour of the night the jailer took them and washed their wounds; then immediately he and all his household were baptized.

Notes

Chapter I: How Did I Get Here?

1. Editorial staff, "Alcohol and Drug Abuse Statistics," American Addiction Centers, last updated March 11, 2022, https://americanaddictioncenters.org/rehab-guide/addiction-statistics.

2. "The State of Pastors 2017: Leading in Complexity," Barna, January 26, 2017, https://www.barna.com/pastors2017/.

3. UHBlog, "The Top 5 Most Stressful Life Events and How to Handle Them," *Healthy@UH* (blog), University Hospitals, July 2, 2015, https://www.uhhospitals.org/Healthy-at-UH /articles/2015/07/the-top-5-most-stressful-life-events.

4. Beth Moore, "Examine How Believers Can Develop Integrity," in *Daniel*, Lifeway, accessed November 11, 2021, https://www.lifeway .com/en/product-family/daniel.

5. *Ghost*, directed by Jerry Zucker (Paramount Pictures, 1990), https://youtu.be/oaX4Ndtutbo.

6. Dr. Henry Cloud and Dr. John Townsend, *Boundaries with Kids: How Healthy Choices Grow Healthy Children* (Grand Rapids: Zondervan, 1998), 72.

Chapter 2: Hiding, Performing, and Pretending

1. "What Is Codependent Personality Disorder?," Family First Intervention, November 9, 2019, https://family-intervention.com/blog/what-is-codependent-personality-disorder/.

2. Pia Mellody, Andrea Wells Miller, and J. Keith Miller, *Facing Codependence: What It Is, Where It Comes From, How It Sabotages Our Lives* (New York: HarperCollins, 2003), 3.

3. Henry Cloud and John Townsend, *Safe People: How to Find Relationships That Are Good for You and Avoid Those That Aren't* (Grand Rapids: Zondervan, 1995), 143.

4. Butler Center for Research, "Why Do People Use Alcohol & Drugs Even After Facing Consequences?," Hazelden Betty Ford Foundation, September 1, 2015, https://www.hazeldenbettyford.org/education/bcr/addiction-research/drug-abuse-brain-ru-915.

5. "The Brain in Recovery: The Neuroscience of Addiction Recovery," Recovery Research Institute, accessed November 11, 2021, https://www.recoveryanswers.org/recovery-101/brain-in-recovery/.

6. Butler Center for Research, "Why Do People Use Alcohol & Drugs?"

7. Brené Brown, "Listening to Shame" (TED Talk, Long Beach Performing Arts Center, Long Beach, CA, March 2, 2012), video shared by TED, on YouTube, March 16, 2012, https://www.youtube.com/watch?v=psN1DORYYV0.

8. John Bradshaw, *Healing the Shame That Binds You*, rev. ed. (Deerfield Beach, FL: Health Communication, 2005).

9. Shirley Davis, "The Neuroscience of Shame," CPTSD Foundation, April 11, 2019, https://cptsdfoundation.org/2019/04/11/the-neuroscience-of-shame/.

10. If you are thinking about suicide or concerned about someone you know committing suicide, stop right now and reach out for help by calling 911, or call the National Suicide Prevention hotline available 24/7 at (800) 273-8255. The website is https://suicidepreventionlifeline.org/.

11. "The 12 Steps of Alcoholics Anonymous (AA)," American

Addiction Centers, updated December 20, 2021, https://www
.alcohol.org/alcoholics-anonymous/.

12. For more information on Celebrate Recovery, visit https/:www
.celebraterecovery.com.

13. James Baldwin, "As Much Truth As One Can Bear," *New York
Times* (book review), January 14, 1962, 38, https://timesmachine.
nytimes.com/timesmachine/1962/01/14/118438007.html?pdf
_redirect=true&auth=login-email&pageNumber=120.

Chapter 3: The Difficult Conversation You're Avoiding

1. *Encyclopaedia Britannica Online*, s.v. "Disease," by Dante G.
Scarpelli, last updated March 6, 2020, https://www.britannica
.com/science/disease.

2. Merriam-Webster, s.v., "addiction," accessed November 15, 2021,
https://www.merriam-webster.com/dictionary/addiction.

3. "The Science of Drug Use and Addiction: The Basics," National
Institute on Drug Abuse, accessed November 12, 2021,
https://www.drugabuse.gov/publications/media-guide/science
-drug-use-addiction-basics.

4. "Understanding Alcohol Use Disorder," National Institute on
Alcohol Abuse and Alcoholism, accessed November 12, 2021,
https://www.niaaa.nih.gov/alcohols-effects-health/alcohol
-use-disorder.

Chapter 4: Reframe Your Story

1. Marjie L. Roddick, "Big T and Little t Trauma and How Your
Body Reacts to It," Good Therapy, October 19, 2015,
www.https://www.goodtherapy.org/blog/big-t-and-little-t
-trauma-and-how-your-body-reacts-to-it-1019154.

2. "Brain Maturity Extends Well Beyond Teen Years," NPR,
October 10, 2011, https://www.npr.org/templates/story/story
.php?storyId=141164708; Sara B. Johnson, Robert W. Blum, Jay
N. Giedd, "Adolescent Maturity and the Brain: The Promise and
Pitfalls of Neuroscience Research in Adolescent Health Policy,"

Journal of Adolescent Health 45, no. 3 (September 2009): 216–21, https://www.ncbi.nlm.nih.gov/pmc/articles/PMC2892678/.

3. "5749. uwd," Bible Hub, accessed November 12, 2021, https://biblehub.com/hebrew/5749.htm.

Chapter 5: Reframe Your Recovery

1. The Free Dictionary, s.v. "recovery," accessed November 12, 2021, https://www.thefreedictionary.com/recovery.

2. "Religious Landscape Study: Women," Pew Research Center, accessed November 12, 2021, https://www.pewforum.org/religious-landscape-study/gender-composition/women/.

3. "Bag Lady," track 12 on Erykah Badu, *Mama's Gun*, Motown Records, 2000.

Chapter 6: Reframe Your Fear

1. "Causes—Post-traumatic Stress Disorder," NHS, accessed November 12, 2021, https://www.nhs.uk/mental-health/conditions/post-traumatic-stress-disorder-ptsd/causes/.

2. "Post-traumatic Stress Disorder: What Is Trauma?" The Center for Treatment of Anxiety and Mood Disorders, accessed November 12, 2021, https://centerforanxietydisorders.com/what-is-trauma/.

3. "Causes—Post-traumatic Stress Disorder."

4. Bessel van der Kolk, *The Body Keeps the Score—Brain, Mind, and Body in the Healing of Trauma* (New York: Viking, 2019), 203.

5. Van der Kolk, 203–4.

6. "Mindfulness STOP Skill," Cognitive Behavioral Therapy Los Angeles, accessed November 12, 2021, https://cogbtherapy.com/mindfulness-meditation-blog/mindfulness-stop-skill.

Chapter 7: Reframe Your Identity

1. Anthony de Mello, *One Minute Wisdom* (New York: Doubleday, 1986; repr. New York: Image, 1988), 97.

2. Ian Morgan Cron and Suzanne Stabile, *The Road Back to You:*

An *Enneagram Journey to Self-Discovery* (Downers Grove, IL: InterVarsity Press, 2016).

3. "Self-Identity Problems," MentalHelp.net, accessed November 12, 2021, https://www.mentalhelp.net/understanding -your-problem/self-identity/.

Chapter 8: Reframe Dysfunction

1. Pia Mellody, Andrea Wells Miller, and J. Keith Miller, *Facing Codependence: What It Is, Where It Comes From, How It Sabotages Our Lives* (New York: HarperCollins, 2003), 107.

2. Dariane Pictet, quoted in Viktoria Memminger, "How Do You Know If You're a Codependent?" Headspace, accessed November 12, 2021, https://www.headspace.com/articles/how -do-you-know-if-youre-a-co-dependent.

3. "Emotional Intelligence in Leadership," Mind Tools, accessed February 2, 2022, https://www.mindtools.com/pages/article /newLDR_45.htm.

4. Jeanne Segal, Melinda Smith, Lawrence Robinson, and Jennifer Shubin, "Improving Emotional Intelligence (EQ)," last updated July 2021, https://www.helpguide.org/articles/mental-health /emotional-intelligence-eq.htm.

5. Peter Scazzero, *Emotionally Healthy Spirituality: Unleash a Revolution in Your Life in Christ* (Nashville: Thomas Nelson, 2006), 17.

6. Peter Scazzero, *The Emotionally Healthy Leader: How Transforming Your Inner Life Will Deeply Transform Your Church, Team, and the World* (Grand Rapids, MI: Zondervan, 2015), 25.

Chapter 9: Reframe Your Normal

1. *Encyclopaedia Britannica Online*, s.v. "Dionysus," by Adam Augustyn, ed., last updated May 26, 2021, https://www.britannica .com/topic/Dionysus.

2. Dr. Karl Benzio, "How Does the Bible Define Alcohol Addiction?," Lighthouse Network, accessed February 3, 2022,

https://lighthousenetwork.org/resources/addictions/alcohol
-rehab-guide/bible-define-alcohol-addiction/.

3. Dictionary.com, s.v. "devotion," accessed November 12, 2021,
   https://www.dictionary.com/browse/devotion.

4. Merriam-Webster, s.v. "devotion," accessed November 12, 2021,
   https://www.merriam-webster.com/dictionary/devotion.

5. J. K. Rowling, "The Fringe Benefits of Failure and the Importance
   of Imagination" (Harvard Commencement Speech, Harvard
   University, Cambridge, MA, June 5, 2008), video shared by
   Harvard University, on YouTube, 12:25, https://www.youtube.com
   /watch?v=UibfDUPJAEU.

6. Amy Morin, "What Is Cognitive Reframing?," Verywell Mind,
   July 30, 2021, https://www.verywellmind.com/reframing-defined
   -2610419.

Chapter 10: The Family Disease

1. Katharina Buchholz, "Substance Abuse Touches Around Half of
   All U.S. Families," November 8, 2019, https://www.statista.com
   /chart/19899/us-families-affected-by-substance-abuse/.

2. The Meadows, "For Families," accessed February 4, 2022,
   https://www.themeadows.com/for-families/.

3. Karen Koenig, quoted in Sara Lindberg, "It's Not Me, It's You:
   Projection Explained in Human Terms," Healthline, updated
   September 15, 2018, https://www.healthline.com/health
   /projection-psychology.

Chapter 11: Holistic Healing

1. "Mindfulness Exercises," Mayo Clinic, accessed November 12, 2021,
   https://www.mayoclinic.org/healthy-lifestyle/consumer-health/in
   -depth/mindfulness-exercises/art-20046356#:~:text=Mindfulness
   %20is%20a%20type%20of,mind%20and%20help%20reduce%20
   stress.

2. "Mindfulness Exercises."

3. Tara Brach, "Feeling Overwhelmed? Remember RAIN,"

Mindful, February 7, 2019, https://www.mindful.org
/tara-brach-rain-mindfulness-practice/.

4. "About Mental Health," Centers for Disease Control and
Prevention, last reviewed June 28, 2021, https://www.cdc.gov
/mentalhealth/learn/index.htm.

5. "What Is EMDR?," EMDR Institute, Inc., accessed
November 12, 2021, https://www.emdr.com/what-is-emdr/.

6. Ariane Resnick, "What Is Somatic Therapy?," Verywell Mind,
updated July 29, 2021, https://www.verywellmind.com/what-is
-somatic-therapy-5190064.

7. "Emotion-Focused Therapy," GoodTherapy, accessed
November 12, 2021, https://www.goodtherapy.org/learn-about
-therapy/types/emotion-focused-therapy.

8. Jodi Clarke, "What Is Imago Therapy?" Verywell Mind, updated
February 9, 2022, https://www.verywellmind.com/imago
-therapy-4172955.

9. "Our Services," CrossRoads Counseling (website), accessed
February 3, 2022, https://www.crossroadscounseling.net/.

10. *Alcoholics Anonymous: The Story of How Many Thousands of Men
and Women Have Recovered from Alcoholism*, 4th ed. (New York:
Alcoholics Anonymous World Services, 2001), 83–84.

Chapter 12: Reframe Your Shame

1. Michelle Graham, *Wanting to Be Her* (Downers Grove, IL:
InterVarsity Press, 2005), 42.

2. "The Neuroscience of Behavior Change," Health Transformer,
August 8, 2017, https://healthtransformer.co/the-neuroscience
-of-behavior-change-bcb567fa83c1.

3. Debbie Ford, "Consciousness Cleanse Day 2: The Gift of Self-
Awareness," Oprah.com, January 5, 2010, https://www.oprah.com
/spirit/consciousness-cleanse-day-2-the-gift-of-self-awareness.

4. Brené Brown, *The Gifts of Imperfection: Let Go of Who You Think
You're Supposed to Be and Embrace Who You Are* (Center City, MN:
Hazelden, 2010), 125.

5. Brené Brown, *I Thought It Was Just Me (But It Isn't): Making the Journey from "What Will People Think?" to "I Am Enough"* (2007; repr., New York: Avery, 2008), 67.

6. "Shame Resilience," Integrative Life Center, February 22, 2021, https://integrativelifecenter.com/wellness-blog/shame-resilience/.

7. Annie Grace, *This Naked Mind: Control Alcohol, Find Freedom, Discover Happiness & Change Your Life* (New York: Avery, 2018).

8. Brené Brown, *Daring Greatly: How the Courage to Be Vulnerable Transforms the Way We Live, Love, Parent, and Lead* (New York: Avery, 2013), 35.

9. "Trust: A Seven-Letter Word," Global Women, August 25, 2020, https://www.globalwomen.org.nz/leadership/trust-a-seven-letter -word/.

10. Maya Angelou, "Dr. Maya Angelou," interview by Oprah, January 2011, MP3 audio, 22:48, episode 35 in *Oprah's Master Class*, OWN, podcast, https://oprahs-master-class-the-podcast .simplecast.com/episodes/dr-maya-angelou-FqtXFBcP.

About the Author

*I*rene Rollins is passionate about the physical, emotional, mental, and spiritual health of people. As a certified emotional intelligence coach, she guides others in becoming the best version of themselves through relatable coaching, teaching, and writing. Irene's fervency to help others overcome their self-defeating habits comes from her own experiences as an overcomer of trauma and alcohol addiction. Irene shares life with her husband, Jimmy Rollins, and her three children: Kayla, Jaden, and Maya. She and Jimmy lead a marriage ministry they founded called TWO=ONE.